Challenges & Choices

Finding Mental Health Services in Ontario

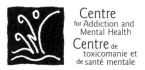

Centre
for Addiction and
Mental Health
Centre de
toxicomanie et
de santé mentale

A Pan American Health Organization /
World Health Organization Collaborating Centre

Challenges & Choices: Finding Mental Health Services in Ontario

National Library of Canada Cataloguing in Publication

Challenges & choices: finding mental health services in Ontario / Centre for Addiction and Mental Health.

ISBN 0-88868-441-X

1. Mental health services—Ontario—Guidebooks. I. Centre for Addiction and Mental Health. II. Title: Challenges and choices.

RA790.7.C3C47 2003   362.2'09713   C2003-900060-5

Product code PR068
Printed in Canada
Copyright © 2003 Centre for Addiction and Mental Health

This book was produced by:

DEVELOPMENT
Margaret Kittel Canale, M.Ed., CAMH

EDITORIAL
Diana Ballon, MSW, CAMH
Kelly Lamorie &
  Megan MacDonald, Double Space

DESIGN
Mara Korkola, MFA, CAMH
Nancy Leung, MFA, CAMH

PRINT PRODUCTION
Christine Harris, CAPPM, CAMH

MARKETING
Arturo Llerenas, MA, CAMH

For information on other Centre for Addiction and Mental Health resource materials or to place an order, please contact:

Marketing and Sales Services
Centre for Addiction and Mental Health
33 Russell Street
Toronto, ON M5S 2S1
Canada

Tel.: 1-800-661-1111 or 416-595-6059 in Toronto
E-mail: marketing@camh.net

Web site: www.camh.net

Disponible en français sous le titre :
Défis et décisions : Trouver des services de santé mentale en Ontario

Acknowledgments

Many people gave their time and expertise to develop this important book. A working group at the Centre for Addiction and Mental Health reviewed several drafts and offered thoughtful feedback. The second and third drafts were reviewed by clients, family members, the general public and service providers across Ontario. This book is the result of their collective wisdom.

For a fuller treatment of this subject, we refer readers to *The Last Taboo: A Survival Guide to Mental Health Care in Canada* by Scott Simmie and Julia Nunes. As well as presenting the opinions of many mental health care providers, this book provides a personal touch and invaluable insight into the mental health system. It is written from the point of view of people who have accessed the system either as a client or family member.

Another useful resource for people living in the Toronto area is *Making Choices: A Consumer/Survivor's Guide to Adult Mental Health Services and Supports in Toronto*. It provides general information as well as many listings for mental health and support services, and is updated regularly.

WRITER
Diana Ballon, MSW, Education and Publishing, CAMH, Toronto

PROJECT MANAGER
Margaret Kittel Canale, M.Ed., Education and Publishing, CAMH, Toronto

CAMH WORKING GROUP

Karyn Baker, MSW, Family Outreach and Response Program, Toronto
Christina Bartha, MSW RSW, Child Psychiatry Program, Toronto
David S. Goldbloom, MD FRCPC, Physician-in-Chief, Toronto
Janice Harris, RN, Emergency Services, Toronto
Elizabeth Hendren-Roberge, M.Sc., Regional Services North, Wawa
Rena Scheffer, Public Education and Information Services, Toronto
Susan Smither, Regional Services Central East, Toronto
Chris Sullivan, Regional Services Central East, Kingston
Ellen Tate, Health Systems Research and Consulting Unit, Toronto
Peter Voore, MD FRCPC, General Psychiatry Program, Toronto

REVIEWERS

Linda Braichet, LPC NCC, Lambton Family Initiative, Sarnia
Robert Buckingham, MD, University Health Network, Toronto
Richard Christie, Centre for Addiction and Mental Health, Kingston
Glen Dewar, Community Resources Consultants of Toronto, Toronto
Teresa Dremetsikas, MD, Canadian Centre for Victims of Torture, Toronto
Randi Fine, MSW, Gerontological Consultant, Toronto
Bill Jesty, Windsor Mood Disorders Self Support Group, Windsor
Anu Lala, B.Sc. DTATI, Women's Health in Women's Hands, Toronto
Karen Liberman, Mood Disorders Association of Ontario, Toronto
Neasa Martin & Associates, Toronto
Ontario Peer Development Initiative, Toronto
Amie Parikh, Centre for Addiction and Mental Health, Toronto
Margaret Pepper, Kettle Point First Nation Health Services, Kettle Point
David Reville & Associates, Toronto
Campbell Thomson, St. Clair Child and Youth Services, Point Edward

We also thank and acknowledge those who reviewed an earlier draft and gave feedback: Peter Chubb, Toronto; Lucy Costa, Toronto; Susan Erdelyan, Windsor; Debby Lessard, Wawa; Dianne Murray, Toronto; Jenn Oakley, Kitchener; Heather Ogilvie, Cornwall; Beth Tiozzo, Cornwall; Patricia Way, Rockland; and Marianne Willars, North Bay.

There are many others who have given us informal feedback and been willing to help whenever we asked for advice. CAMH staff include Gail Czukar, general counsel; Brian McLean and Anita Persaud, Community Support and Research Unit; Wendy Nailer and Diana Musson, Work Adjustment and Employment Support Services; Wayne Skinner, Concurrent Disorders Program; and Wende Wood, Department of Pharmaceutical Services. And thanks to Lora Patton, legal counsel for the Psychiatric Patient Advocate Office.

Table of Contents

2003 Centre for Addiction & Mental Health

Note to service providers

Service providers surveyed about their need for public mental health information indicated they lacked information about mental health services in Ontario for clients and families. Thus the idea for *Challenges & Choices: Finding Mental Health Services in Ontario* was conceived.

While this guide is written in plain language and directed to clients and families, you, as service providers, will no doubt find this information useful—both for your own background knowledge, and to share with clients and families. The size of the pages and the binding were selected specifically to make it easy for you to photocopy sections of the book for clients. You may also want to keep a copy of the book in your waiting room, or have it as a reference guide for people coming to your office. Regardless, our primary goal is to see that as many people as possible benefit from the information in this book.

Actual production of the guide took close to a year. It was reviewed extensively by a working group at the Centre for Addiction and Mental Health; by experts working at various mental health agencies and organizations across the province; and through interviews with clients, family members and the general public. Reviewers represented a broad range of backgrounds; for example, they come from rural and urban areas across Ontario and from diverse ethnocultural and racial groups. And they have varying experiences and expertise.

We hope you and the clients you share this with find it to be a helpful resource.

About
the guide

Who is the guide for?

This guide is for people looking for mental health services in Ontario. You could be looking for services for yourself, a family member, partner or friend. Or you could be a health care provider who wants to help clients and families find out about different services and how to use them.

How do I use the guide?

The range of services you are seeking will vary, depending on your situation. You could be trying to find a therapist to help you deal with the CHALLENGES of a small or minor difficulty, or you could be coping with a severe and ongoing mental health problem.

This guide is really about CHOICES. It provides information about mental health services available in Ontario to help you choose what's best for you. It also offers a brief description of some of the most common types of mental health problems. And it gives tips that will help you find the services you need. It provides phone numbers and Web site addresses, so you can research a specific problem or treatment in more detail. And it includes questions you can ask health care providers. These questions can help you make sure that you're getting the kind of care you want.

Whether services are available will depend on where you live and the type of services you need. People living in large cities, for example, will have access to many services. However, services will be limited in smaller urban centres and perhaps non-existent in rural areas. The same is basically true if you are seeking services that are sensitive to age, gender and gender identity, sexual orientation, race, culture, ethnicity, religion, ability, income or education. You may have to shop around for services that suit your particular wants and needs. If the services you need are too far away, for instance, you may need to use services close by, even if they are not as specialized.

Some sections of this guide will be important for you while others may not relate to your concerns or the kind of help you are seeking. Use the table of contents to find the sections that will be most helpful for you.

If you are a health care provider, you may want to use *Challenges & Choices* as a reference book for clients. Feel free to photocopy sections that you think might be helpful for your clients. The size and format of the book were especially designed for this purpose. If you have a copy of the book in your waiting room, clients will be able to browse through the sections, and let you know which parts they would like copied.

We know that people have different beliefs about what mental health problems are. And people have different ideas about how to deal with these problems. This guide will be useful in outlining what's available. But you should make the final decisions about what services are right for you.

Because this is a guide for people in Ontario, we mainly list resources that can be used by people living anywhere in the province. You can keep track of contact information for services in your area by listing them in Appendix D, a blank page at the back of the book.

A word about language

In the mental health field, many different words are used to describe the same thing. However, these words don't always reflect all cultures or ways of looking at a problem. People from some cultures have no words to define mental health problems. And some cultures may see certain behaviours as positive that others see as problems. In this guide, we use words that are commonly understood to be the most respectful.

Instead of saying that people have a mental illness, we prefer to say that people are seeking services for mental health problems. Sometimes when we describe different types of mental health problems, we use the word "disorder," as this is the word the medical profession uses in its diagnoses of clients.

In referring to people with a certain mental health problem, we speak of people with schizophrenia, for example, rather than saying that a person is "schizophrenic." We use the term "people with" because people are people first and shouldn't be labelled or identified by their challenges.

Sometimes we describe people who use mental health services as "clients." However, we recognize that there are many different terms for people using these services. What one person prefers may be quite different from what someone else likes. Other terms sometimes used are "user," "patient," "consumer" or "survivor." (In Section 13: Understanding Your Rights, we use "patient" because the Ontario *Mental Health Act* uses that word.)

When we use the term "family member," we are referring to someone who has a relative, partner or close friend with a mental health problem.

Introduction

1

One in five people in Ontario has a mental health problem at some point in his or her life. Only about 30 per cent of these people seek any kind of help. There are several reasons for this. People may not recognize that they have a problem. They may not know what kind of help is available. Or they may know what exists but not be able to use the services because of barriers, such as cost, language and transportation. And they may have difficulty finding what they want when there is a wide range of services, and no one place to access them. In some cases, there won't be the right services nearby for their specific concerns.

Still others may know they have a problem but don't seek help because of the stigma (prejudice and discrimination) attached to mental health problems. They feel embarrassed or ashamed. They worry about being discriminated against. They worry that they will be judged, misunderstood and perhaps left out because of their difficulties. When people feel discriminated against, it's harder for them to seek help. Sometimes they don't acknowledge a problem for which they could get treatment. This is unfortunate because there *are* services that can help. And the earlier someone gets help, the less chance there is of the problem coming back or getting worse.

1

CHALLENGE: The fear of being discriminated against for having a mental health problem may be preventing you from seeking help. For instance, you may fear that someone will deny you services, not include you or treat you differently if they know you have a mental health problem.

SUGGESTIONS: Mental health providers have to keep your personal information confidential: expect privacy from them. Telephone help lines and self-help groups are examples of some of the confidential services available.

Consider confiding in someone you feel that you can trust. This person should understand your situation and be willing to support you. How you communicate what you are experiencing is your choice. Some people believe that to reduce stigma or prejudice against people with mental health problems, it's important to talk about the challenges they face openly. But some people have been discriminated against because they openly talk about their challenges in the workplace or in other social situations.

While you don't want to create stigma by hiding a mental health problem, sometimes it's important to protect yourself. For instance, if you live in a small town, you may want to consider using a mental health agency or hospital somewhere else.

Mental health problems are common. So if you are experiencing difficulties, know that you are not alone.

You can feel better, and you may even fully recover. But mental health problems can take time to work through. It's important to focus on your abilities and strengths. Allow yourself opportunities to heal.

Finding your way around the mental health system can be confusing, frustrating, scary—and difficult. That's why we've created this guide. In it, we tell you the basics about the most common mental health problems. We give information about the services available—from hospital treatment to community support. We explain a bit about the kinds of people who provide the care. And we summarize mental health laws, so that you will know your rights and how you can make best use of the system.

For family and friends who want to help but don't know how, this guide outlines ways they can access the system for you. In the process, they can learn how to take care of themselves as well.

Take charge of your situation by being actively involved in your care. When you meet with a health care provider or go to a certain agency, decide whether the support they offer is what you want and need. Help to shape your treatment by suggesting what has worked for you in the past. If you're not happy with the services offered, let them know. You can also suggest how the services could be improved. If it's possible, you might want to find services somewhere else.

Q&A **QUESTION:** Isn't it easier to just work out my problems on my own?

ANSWER: That's like saying you can deal with a heart condition or any other physical problem without help from a doctor. Mental health problems are as valid a reason as physical health problems for getting help. Without support or treatment, mental health problems can get worse. Looking for help is a sign of strength, not weakness. It shows that you know there is a problem and are taking steps to address it.

Knowledge is power

You may know that you have a problem but not know exactly what it is. Recognizing a problem is the first step toward solving it. The next step is to find the kind of services that will best meet your needs.

Start by getting as much information as you can about your symptoms and the supports available to help you. The more you know, the better decisions you will make. And the more power and control you will have to deal with the situation. Keep in mind that you might have to go to various sources before you find the information you need.

1

Getting information you need may mean:

- talking to people you know
- going to a public library
- going through the phone book and finding a mental health agency or clinic that you can call (See Appendix B for a list of organizations in Ontario that deal with mental health problems.)
- going to a bookstore and looking in the health/self-help section
- checking the Internet: you can search the Internet by using key words like "mental health," "psychotherapy" or "mental illness." You can also type in the kind of problem you want to know more about plus "services." (Keep in mind that not all information on the Internet is correct.) In Appendix B, we include some recommended Web sites. (If you don't have a computer or access to the Internet, public libraries or community agencies often do.)
- going to educational groups or sessions organized through support or self-help groups, hospitals, community agencies or other organizations. These groups can help you recognize and learn how to manage mental health problems or better understand a mental health issue. Through the process, you can talk about how it feels to live and cope with a new diagnosis or difficulty. Talking openly about your feelings will often help you deal with the situation better. It will also help you decide on a treatment plan that makes sense to you.

You should be aware that the mental health system in North America tends to be based on what is referred to as the "medical model." The medical model tends to see a mental health problem as an illness or disease requiring medication and/or psychotherapy. Medication is used to change biochemical processes in the brain that are believed to contribute to the mental health problem.

There is a gradual move toward a more community-based psychosocial rehabilitation model. This is a model that helps people who have a mental health problem gain or relearn skills they need to live in the community and cope with their difficulties. It addresses a variety of areas, including housing, basic skills training, employment and social supports and living skills (e.g., cooking, shopping, budgeting, using transportation).

CHALLENGE: There is a shortage of services in languages other than English.

SUGGESTIONS: Find out if the agency has cultural interpreters. Or bring someone with you who can interpret. Check to see if they have information pamphlets and phone lines in different languages.

You may also want to seek spiritual support from someone in your own community, such as a spiritual adviser who speaks the same language as you and understands your culture.

About mental health and mental health problems

2

What is mental health?

Mental health involves finding a balance in all aspects of your life: physically, mentally, emotionally and spiritually. It is the ability to enjoy life and deal with the challenges you face every day—whether that involves making choices and decisions, adapting to and coping in difficult situations or talking about your needs and desires.

Just as your life and circumstances continually change, so do your moods and thoughts, and your sense of well-being. It's important to find balance in your life over time and in a range of situations. It's natural to feel off balance at times: for example, sad, worried, scared or suspicious. But these kinds of feelings may become a problem if they get in the way of your daily life over a long period.

What contributes to mental health problems?

There are many beliefs about why people have mental health problems. Scientific studies suggest that many serious mental health problems involve biochemical disturbances in the brain. Professionals also believe that various psychological, social and environmental factors affect your well-being. As well, mental health is affected by the physical, mental, emotional and spiritual parts of your life. Stress can affect how you cope in any or all of these areas and can make it harder to manage day-to-day activities. You may have difficulty coping because you lack new skills and information that could help you.

You may be struggling with such difficulties as:

2

- going through a divorce
- dealing with the death of a loved one
- having a car accident
- coping with a physical health problem
- growing up in a war-torn country, leaving the country you came from or adjusting to a new country (which often means dealing with immigration and resettlement experiences)
- dealing with racism or other forms of prejudice (because of sexual orientation, age, religion, culture, class, etc.)
- having a low income or being homeless
- not having equal access to education, work and health care
- having a history of mental health problems in the family or
- being a victim of violence, abuse or other trauma.

Your mental health can also be affected by how much love, support and acceptance you receive from family and others.

It is important to know that not all cultures view mental health in the same way. For example, in some countries, people who have schizophrenia are seen as having special powers and insights.

Alcohol and other drug use do not usually cause a mental health problem. However, they are often used to help cope with the problem. And they can make the mental health problem worse.

You and your health care provider need to work together to identify the problem, what may have caused or contributed to your difficulties and how you can be helped. Whatever the cause, you should know that mental health problems are not your fault. No one chooses to have a problem.

Types of mental health problems

Mental health problems often take different shapes and forms at different times.

Some people feel depressed. Others feel anxious and fearful. A child might act out in class or avoid others. Some don't eat much. Others overeat. Some depend on alcohol or other drugs to numb their painful feelings. Still others lose touch with reality. For example, they may hear voices, see things that aren't there or believe things that aren't true. Some have suicidal thoughts—and some act on these thoughts. Some feel angry and aggressive. And some people are traumatized because of a single event, such as a serious car accident, or because of a more long-term problem, such as years of being abused as a child. Many people have more than one of these problems at a time.

For many years, we thought mental health problems would either keep coming back or would never go away. We now know that many people recover from these challenges. Many people with mental health problems get better by using their own strength and resilience, the support of family and friends, psychotherapy, techniques to lessen their stress and possibly medication.

In the next section, we will be using the term "disorder" to describe some of the most common mental health problems and labels used by the medical profession in making a diagnosis.

Some people may be relieved to know how doctors identify their problems. They may be glad to get a diagnosis that provides a theory about what's wrong and suggestions for how their problems could be treated. But others may not find it helpful to know a diagnosis. They may see it as a label or category that doesn't describe their situation. Or they may believe that their condition is due to difficult life situations rather than an illness.

In truth, some people are wrongly diagnosed and then given the wrong kind of treatment. Sometimes their mental health diagnosis changes so many times over the years that they lose confidence in the system. However, others find that an accurate diagnosis helps them choose the right treatment and results in the best care.

2

Here are some common diagnoses:

Anxiety disorders are believed to be the most common mental health problem in North America, particularly among people who are depressed. In fact, as many as two-thirds of the people who have depression also have strong symptoms of anxiety. While we all feel anxious from time to time, "anxiety" refers to excessive worrying that is hard to control. People who experience anxiety feel restless or "keyed up" and on edge. They may get tired easily or feel their minds going blank. They may also feel irritated, have tense muscles, trouble concentrating and sleep problems.

The main types of anxiety disorders are panic disorder, obsessive-compulsive disorder (OCD), post-traumatic stress disorder (PTSD), generalized anxiety disorder (GAD) and social and specific phobias.

> For more information on anxiety disorders, contact the Anxiety Disorders Association of Ontario at (613) 729-6761 in Ottawa or toll-free at 1-877-308-3843. Or view their Web site at www.anxietyontario.com. For more information on OCD, call the Ontario Obsessive Compulsive Disorder Network at (416) 410-4772 in Toronto or view their Web site at www.oocdn.org.

Attention-deficit/hyperactivity disorder (ADHD) is one of the main reasons why children are referred for mental health services. ADHD affects a child's attention span and concentration. It can also affect how impulsive and active the child is. The energetic way in which children normally behave shouldn't be confused with symptoms of ADHD. Children who have ADHD are much more active, distracted, persistent and impulsive than other children. Symptoms of ADHD persist over time.

An Ontario study predicts that five to nine per cent of school-aged children may have ADHD. ADHD is three to four times more common in boys than girls. About two-thirds of children with ADHD continue to have the symptoms in adolescence.

2

ADHD is less common in adults. Adults with ADHD may be easily distracted (e.g., continually bored, forgetful or anxious). They may also be depressed, have low self-esteem, mood swings and difficulties at work and at other activities.

Bipolar disorder was previously known as manic-depressive illness. It involves extreme mood swings that may have nothing to do with what's going on in the person's life. Typically, people with bipolar disorder move between feeling very low or depressed and feeling very high or "manic." When people are manic, they may take part in risky and unusual activities, increase sexual behaviours or get in trouble with the law. They may also feel invincible or all-powerful, have racing thoughts and other symptoms. There's a good chance that people with bipolar disorder will feel "normal" and function well at times too. How long the episodes last and how often they occur will vary, depending on the person.

People often experience the first sign of a problem in adolescence or early adulthood. It may begin with an episode of depression and not be followed by a manic episode for several years. Women may have symptoms when they are pregnant, or shortly after. Overall, men and women are affected equally.

> For more information, contact the Mood Disorders Association of Ontario (MDAO) at (416) 486-8046 in Toronto or toll-free at 1-888-486-8236. Or view their Web site at www.mooddisorders.on.ca.

Conduct disorders involve behavioural and emotional difficulties. Children and youth with a conduct disorder find it difficult to follow rules and behave in a socially acceptable way. They may cause property loss or damage, steal or lie, seriously violate rules or be violent toward other people or animals. While conduct disorders are the most common psychiatric diagnoses among children, the disorders can be present at any age.

2

For more information, view the section related to conduct disorders at the Web site of the American Academy of Child & Adolescent Psychiatry at www.aacap.org/publications/factsfam/conduct.htm.

Depression is more than simply being unhappy. Someone who is depressed feels abnormally sad, despairing and hopeless in a sustained way for more than two weeks. Depression may impair how the person performs at work, school and in relationships. The person's sleep, energy, appetite, concentration, memory and sexual desire may also be affected. The person may lose interest or pleasure in life, feel irritable, worthless or guilty and, in some cases, may think of suicide.

Women are diagnosed with depression twice as often as men are. There are many theories about why this is true. One theory is that women seek health care services more often than men. Life and body changes may also play a part: women are more likely to become depressed after puberty, during their menstrual cycles and following pregnancy. Another theory is that women have less power and control in their lives, and are more likely to be victims of violence or abuse.

While women are more frequently diagnosed with depression, a rising number of men are also seeking treatment. Men may use substances, such as alcohol or other drugs, to cope. These drugs may hide their feelings of depression.

Other factors can also contribute to depression, such as prejudice and discrimination and being marginalized or excluded. This may mean being denied your rights, not being recognized or appreciated and not being allowed to participate in things that are important to you.

Often, people of colour, older adults, lesbians, gays, bisexuals and transgendered people are affected by discrimination. People who have suffered major losses may also be more at risk of having depression.

> For more information about depression, contact the Mood Disorders Association of Ontario (MDAO) at (416) 486-8046 in Toronto or toll-free at 1-888-486-8236. Or view their Web site at www.mooddisorders.on.ca

Eating disorders are a range of conditions involving an obsession with food, weight and appearance. This obsession negatively affects people's health, relationships and day-to-day living. The two main types of eating disorders are anorexia nervosa and bulimia nervosa.

People with anorexia have an intense and irrational fear of gaining weight and having body fat. They are obsessed with being thin. They may believe they are fat, even when they are well below the normal weight for their height and age.

People with bulimia go through cycles of bingeing and purging. Bingeing involves eating large amounts of food quickly. This makes people feel physically ill and anxious about gaining weight. Then they will purge, which can involve vomiting, depriving themselves of food, overexercising or using laxatives and diuretics.

About 90 per cent of people diagnosed with eating disorders are girls and women. However, these days boys are being diagnosed with eating problems more often. These disorders typically begin during adolescence.

> For more information, contact the National Eating Disorder Information Centre at (416) 340-4156 in Toronto or toll-free at 1-866-633-4220. Or view their Web site at www.nedic.ca.

People who have a **personality disorder** behave and communicate in ways that are very different from what is expected in the society they live in. They may have problems with self-image or having successful relationships. They may have a different way of seeing themselves, others and the world. And they may have a rigid way of thinking, feeling and acting. This makes it difficult for them to get used to changes and stresses that are an unavoidable part of everyday living.

2

While personality disorders may look different in different people, anyone who has a personality disorder deals with feeling uncomfortable with themselves or others. Personality disorders begin in adolescence or early adulthood. Some personality disorders may result from childhood sexual or physical trauma.

Schizophrenia affects all aspects of a person's functioning—how he or she feels, thinks, acts and relates to others. People with schizophrenia often have difficulty figuring out what is real and what is fantasy. For instance, they may see or hear things that aren't actually there. They may also have difficulty carrying out everyday tasks such as bathing, getting dressed and preparing simple meals.

Men and women are both affected equally by schizophrenia. However, men tend to experience their first episode in their late teens or early 20s. Women may not experience symptoms until they are a few years older.

> For more information about schizophrenia, contact the Schizophrenia Society
> of Canada at (905) 415-2007 in Toronto or toll-free at 1-888-SSC-HOPE
> (772-4673). Or view their Web site at www.schizophrenia.ca. You can
> also contact the Schizophrenia Society of Ontario at (416) 449-6830 in
> Toronto, toll-free at 1-800-449-6367, or through their Web site at
> www.schizophrenia.on.ca.

Substance use disorders involve dependence on or abuse of substances, such as alcohol, medication or illegal drugs. Most people who use substances do not progress to problem use or become dependent on substances. But those who do develop a substance use problem are at high risk of having a mental health problem as well. For instance, people with anxiety, depression or conduct disorders or those who have a history of child abuse may use alcohol or other drugs to help them cope (e.g., to feel more calm or less worried) and then become addicted to the substance. Sometimes substance use hides the mental health problem, so the problem does not get addressed.

Some drugs—such as alcohol, sedatives (to help people sleep or feel less anxious), stimulants or "uppers" (that make people feel they have more energy) and marijuana—can lead to depression, anxiety or psychosis (e.g., schizophrenia, bipolar disorder). Often these problems will go away when the person stops using the substances.

When someone has both a substance use and mental health problem, they have what is called a concurrent disorder. Like mental health problems, substance use problems affect how poeple think, behave and relate with others. They also affect people's interests and performance in school or work.

> Descriptions of these mental health problems can be downloaded from the Canadian Mental Health Association (CMHA), Ontario Division Web site at www.ontario.cmha.ca and from the Web site of the National Institute of Mental Health at www.nimh.nih.gov.
>
> To get a more detailed description of these mental health problems and information about others not listed here, contact the Centre for Addiction and Mental Health (CAMH)'s 24-hour information line at (416) 595-6111 in Toronto or toll-free at 1-800-463-6273.
>
> For a small charge, you can obtain booklets on obsessive-compulsive disorder (a type of anxiety disorder), depression, bipolar disorder and schizophrenia by contacting CAMH's Marketing and Sales Services at (416) 595-6059 in Toronto or toll-free at 1-800-661-1111.
>
> Contact the Ontario Drug and Alcohol Registry of Treatment (DART) for up-to-date details about alcohol and other drug treatment services across the province. Their toll-free number is 1-800-565-8603. Their Web site is www.dart.on.ca.

Getting an assessment

3

You may decide to talk to a co-worker, friend or a spiritual adviser about a mental health difficulty, without formally using the mental health system. But if you do decide you want to use the services available, you will likely need to have an assessment. This evaluation will help identify the types of difficulties you are having. It will also help determine the kind of services you think would be helpful.

General practitioners, psychiatrists and psychologists are the only health care providers who can give an official diagnosis. These professionals should explain the diagnosis, the kind of treatment being suggested and the reasons for this type of treatment. (If they don't explain, make sure you ask them their opinion before you leave the office.)

Other health care professionals, such as nurses or social workers, can assess your situation but can't make a diagnosis.

QUESTION: Do I need a diagnosis to get treatment?

ANSWER: You don't necessarily need a diagnosis to get treatment. However, it may be helpful to get a thorough assessment and diagnosis to help direct your treatment. If you have information about your condition, you'll have a better idea, for instance, if you need medication, or if there is a certain kind of therapy that would be most helpful.

But even if you get a diagnosis, it may change or be interpreted differently, depending on the doctor who is assessing you. Some conditions are difficult to diagnose, and sometimes the only way to figure out what you are dealing with is to see how the condition develops over time. Assessments usually involve a conversation with your health care provider. Sometimes you'll need to fill out a questionnaire.

3

During an assessment, you will likely discuss things such as:

- why you have come for help, what kind of help you are looking for and what has helped in the past
- what condition you are in physically
- what problems you have been having, and how long they have lasted
- whether you've had recent stresses, such as a sudden change or loss (e.g., a death, losing a job)
- if you've experienced or seen violence (e.g., physical or sexual assault, war), even if it occurred years before
- if there is a history of mental health problems in your family
- what your life is like: how you feel, what you think, how you sleep, if you exercise and socialize, how you do at school or work, how your relationships with friends and family are
- if you've come to Canada in the last few years, and/or if you've come from a war-torn country
- what, if any, medications you are taking and
- any other topics you would like to discuss.

Assessments can go many ways. You may decide you simply need more support during stressful times. You may need to find affordable housing. You may need to find meaningful work and adequate pay. Or the person giving the assessment may recommend that you see a therapist or that you start taking medication. He or she could also encourage you to seek other types of services.

Where to go for an assessment

FAMILY DOCTORS/GENERAL PRACTITIONERS

Family doctors, or general practitioners (GPs), are often the first professionals that people talk to about a mental health problem. In fact, family doctors spend up to half their time identifying and treating mental health problems. Doctors are able to examine your physical health and rule out problems that could be adding to or affecting changes in your mood, thinking or behaviour. They may ask some questions about your symptoms and what kind of stress you are coping with.

Sometimes doctors can do a full psychiatric assessment, particularly for the more common conditions, such as depression or anxiety. Other times, doctors will suggest that you see a psychiatrist, because psychiatrists have specialized training in identifying and treating mental health problems.

COMMUNITY AGENCIES

Community agencies can also offer assessments. The type of assessment will depend on the health care provider available. Sometimes this may be a doctor, psychologist, social worker or nurse. But in smaller cities and rural areas, you are more likely to be seen by a community mental health worker. This person will match your needs with the services available at the agency.

Social workers and community mental health workers tend to focus on the social situation that may be affecting your mental health (e.g., poverty, family situation, work, support systems, if you have violence in your life). They also examine what supports you need to cope or manage better in the community. If you have a serious mental health problem, you will likely also need to see someone who is medically trained, such as a family doctor or preferably a psychiatrist. This doctor will assess your need for medication or other medical help.

PSYCHIATRISTS

Even if you believe you've identified your problem after reading or hearing a description of it, it's a good idea to get an assessment from a psychiatrist. Family doctors often have a list of psychiatrists they can refer you to. (Psychiatrists almost always need a referral from a doctor before they can see you.) After you book an appointment, you may have to wait about two to three months to see a psychiatrist. *(To find a psychiatrist, see p. 31 on family doctors/general practitioners. This section describes how to find a psychiatrist as well as a doctor.)*

QUESTION: My psychiatrist said that I have X diagnosis, but I don't agree. What should I do?

ANSWER: If you don't agree with your diagnosis, you should ask your family doctor to refer you to another psychiatrist for a second opinion. People often don't ask for a second opinion because they don't want to offend their doctor. But in reality, most doctors are open to their clients seeking another perspective and may even suggest it themselves.

Remember, it's your health, and you have the right to get another opinion.

For more information on specific types of disorders, contact the Canadian Mental Health Association (CMHA), Ontario Division. Descriptions of these disorders can be downloaded from their Web site at www.ontario.cmha.ca.

EMERGENCY DEPARTMENTS OF HOSPITALS

If you are in a crisis or can't wait for an appointment, go to the emergency department of a nearby hospital. But be prepared for a long wait! You may want to bring someone to keep you company who can help look out for your best interests.

You will first be seen by a nurse. If the nurse determines that there is concern for your safety, you will then be seen by the emergency room doctor. Based on his or her assessment, the doctor has three options, to:

1. release you
2. refer you to a mental health professional or
3. admit you to the hospital.

3

If the situation does not require immediate medical care, the next step may be for you to get a more in-depth assessment from a crisis worker. This person is often a nurse or social worker. If the worker thinks that you will be able to manage safely out of hospital, he or she may direct you to outpatient or crisis services. The crisis worker may set up an appointment with you for a couple of days later to see how you're doing.

CHALLENGE: There are few, if any, mental health services in my community.

SUGGESTIONS: In areas that don't have many services, you will probably be referred by your family doctor to a local hospital or health centre. If there are no psychiatrists on staff at the hospital or centre, you may be seen by a visiting psychiatrist.

Videoconferencing is another way to get an assessment. It allows you to benefit from the expertise of a professional not in your area, without either of you having to travel.

If you don't have a family doctor, you can go to the emergency department of the nearest hospital.

About
therapy

4

The right help for you will depend on a number of factors, including:

- the mental health problem(s) you are facing
- the seriousness of the problem, and whether you need help for a short or long period
- your understanding of how to improve your state of mind
- what is available where you live and your ability to travel (e.g., in terms of cost and time), if there are no services close to your home
- your spiritual values and beliefs
- whether your therapist is able to respect personal characteristics, such as your age, gender, sexual orientation, religion, race, cultural and ethnic background, ability and income, and is able to respond to your needs
- the type of care that you feel most comfortable with.
- the language you speak, and your therapist's ability to communicate and work with you.
- whether you can afford to pay for therapy.

One type of treatment or one type of therapist may not always be able to provide you with everything you need. For instance, you may visit a spiritual adviser to talk about difficulties you are having. You may see a psychiatrist for a medication prescription. You may go to yoga or exercise classes to help you relax and feel less stressed. You may see a nutritionist to help you explore how various foods can influence your mood or thinking. Or you may find it useful to talk with your family doctor or a friend.

People go to psychotherapists to discuss the problems they have identified. They may get therapy one-on-one, as part of a couple, family or group. There is scientific research proving the effectiveness of both medication and psychotherapy to treat mental health problems, as well as proof of their effectiveness when used together.

QUESTION: How do I know when a problem is serious enough that I should find professional help?

ANSWER: It depends on the person. Generally, people seek professional help when their problem is really interfering with their lives (e.g., relationships, work, school) and their ability to function and enjoy themselves.

Choosing a therapist

Psychotherapists are mental health professionals who use "talking therapy" or counselling to help people with things such as self-esteem, changing beliefs and ways of thinking, communication and relationship skills and working through difficult issues from the past. People generally see psychotherapists when their problems affect their day-to-day living. These problems may be negatively influencing their work or school, their relationships and their ability to enjoy life. A psychotherapist can offer support, help you better understand your problems and help you learn new ways of coping.

If you're looking for a therapist, you can ask:

- your family doctor
- a nurse
- a community mental health worker
- a social work or outpatient psychiatric department of a hospital
- an employee (and family) assistance program through your work

- a religious or spiritual leader or organization
- a community information centre
- a social service agency (e.g., mental health association) or
- a self-help group.

Often the best way to find a therapist is to get a recommendation from a friend, family member or a health care provider whose opinion you respect. When you do get referrals, try to get more than one at a time, and get on several waiting lists, if necessary.

QUESTION: How can talking to a therapist help me deal with my problems? Isn't it just as good to talk to a friend whom I already trust?

ANSWER: In some cases, speaking to a friend who will listen and be supportive may be enough. However, if your problem persists, it may be helpful to speak to someone who isn't connected to your life — someone who can offer a safe and neutral point of view. Therapists offer the advantage of being trained and having practice talking in ways that have proven helpful.

Interviewing a therapist

Don't be afraid to ask therapists questions to find out if you are comfortable with their style and approach. Below are some sample questions.

- What educational and professional training do you have?
- How many years of experience do you have working as a therapist?
- Do you have specific training or experience working with my particular issue (e.g., trauma, divorce, childhood sexual abuse)?
- What is your approach to therapy for my specific problem?
- Are you a member of an association or professional organization?

You may want to consider whether you want a therapist of the same gender, sexual orientation or ethnic background as you. There may also be other characteristics that you want your therapist to have in common with you, or to at least be sensitive to (e.g., issues of race, culture, age) or other factors that you see as important to your identity and way of viewing the world. As well, it's a good idea to find out how many sessions the therapist will provide and how much the therapy will cost. *(See How much will therapy cost?, p. 35.)*

QUESTION: What if I'm not comfortable with my therapist or with how the therapy is working?

ANSWER: A trusting relationship between you and the therapist is key to successful therapy. If you are feeling uncomfortable with your therapist, it's possible that your personalities may not be the right fit. Or the therapist may be offering a form of therapy that is not useful to you. However, it's equally possible that your discomfort could be related to bringing a difficult issue out into the open or the anxiety of speaking to someone new.

To determine the source of your discomfort, it's important to discuss your concerns with your therapist. If you have had therapy before, it's also useful to tell your therapist what worked and what didn't work with other therapists. This will give your new therapist an idea of what you want from the therapy and if he or she can provide it.

But don't stick around in therapy if it's not working. You can fire your therapist! But if you do, make sure that there is someone else who will be able to see you. Your therapist may be able to refer you to another therapist.

Note: It is not ethical for a therapist to see you outside of therapy. It is not right for the therapist to be your friend or for you to end up giving therapy to the therapist! And it is WRONG for a therapist to make any type of sexual comments or to behave sexually. If you have any concerns about your therapist, call his or her governing or regulatory college and tell them what happened.

There are many different types of therapists who vary in the amount and type of training they've received. Following are some of the more common types.

Types of therapists

FAMILY DOCTORS/GENERAL PRACTITIONERS

Family doctors, or general practitioners (GPs), are often the first health care professionals someone will turn to when they have a mental health problem. A family doctor may prescribe medication, talk briefly to you about your concerns or refer you to a mental health specialist. Some general practitioners offer psychotherapy as a full-time practice.

General practitioners don't receive much psychotherapy training as part of their general medical degree. So it's important to ask them if they had additional training in psychotherapy after completing medical school. Therapy from a general practitioner or family doctor is covered by OHIP. Doctors who call themselves a "GP psychotherapist" have a special interest in psychotherapy. However, they aren't required to have additional training to be part of their professional organization, the GP Psychotherapy Association.

> To find a family doctor in your area, you can call the Find a Doctor service available through the College of Physicians and Surgeons of Ontario at (416) 967-2626 in Toronto or toll-free at 1-800-268-7096. Or view their Web site at www.cpso.on.ca.
>
> To get a referral to a GP psychotherapist, call the GP Psychotherapy Association at (416) 410-6644 in Toronto.

PSYCHIATRISTS

Psychiatrists have a medical degree and five years of psychiatric training. Because psychiatrists are medical doctors, they are licensed to prescribe medication and provide psychotherapy. Their services are covered by OHIP. As medical doctors, they are more likely to identify connections between psychiatric and physical health problems. Some clients report that psychiatrists tend to be more focused on medication than on talking therapy—perhaps because of their medical training. However, some psychiatrists put emphasis on psychotherapy in their practice.

It is often very difficult to find a psychiatrist who is available to see you without a long wait, particularly if you live outside a large city. In fact, in some underserviced communities, there may not be a psychiatrist on staff at the nearest hospital. These hospitals instead rely on visiting psychiatrists from larger cities or videoconferencing. Through videoconferencing, psychiatrists are able to assess and follow up with clients even though they are in different locations.

If psychiatrists are not available, psychiatric residents (medical doctors who are in training to become psychiatrists) may be available. Residents spend at least five years training to become a psychiatrist after they graduate from medical school. The work they do as psychotherapists is closely supervised by staff.

> To find a psychiatrist in your area, you can call the Find a Doctor service
> listed above under Family doctors/General practitioners. You can also get
> a referral from your family doctor or visit an outpatient psychiatric clinic.

PSYCHOLOGISTS

Psychologists have at least nine years of university education. They also have at least one year of supervised practice. To be able to register with the College of Psychologists of Ontario, psychologists must pass oral and written exams. They have a lot of training in doing assessments, which includes making diagnoses and providing therapy. Psychologists have a PhD or PsyD, but their fees are not covered by OHIP, and they cannot prescribe medication. However, the services they provide through hospitals, community agencies or private clinics or offices may be available without charge. Their fees may also be partly covered under extended health insurance plans, the Workplace Safety and Insurance Board (WSIB) or other private insurance programs.

> To get a referral to a psychologist in your area, ask your family doctor or call the Ontario Psychological Association at (416) 961-0069 in Toronto or toll-free at 1-800-268-0069. The association will provide names of psychologists in private practice in your area. They can also provide details about the services they offer, the language they are offered in and the focus of their work (e.g., eating disorders, family violence, learning disability assessments).

4

OTHER HEALTH CARE PROFESSIONALS

Professionals from a variety of other fields (e.g., social work, nursing, occupational therapy) may also provide therapy. Depending on the field, their training may range from a diploma to a PhD. Many of these professionals supplement their education by taking extra courses and counselling training from universities or hospitals. Some take advantage of community-based workshops, training programs, seminars and conferences.

Social workers and nurses are particularly common in a psychiatric setting. They also tend to be available more often than doctors. Social workers are trained to focus on how a person's social environment affects his or her health. (By social environment, we're referring to a person's housing, family, work, financial situations, social supports, education, gender, etc.) *(See How much will therapy cost, p. 35.)*

> To get a referral to a social worker in private practice, you can call the Ontario Association of Social Workers at (416) 923-4848 in Toronto or view their Web site at www.oasw.org. The association will try to match you with three social workers from the age group (e.g., child, adolescent), specialty (e.g., marital counselling) and language you desire.

QUESTION: Is what I say to my therapist private and confidential?

ANSWER: Trust is the basis of a good relationship. Part of this trust involves knowing that what you say to your therapist will be kept between the two of you. Therapists must keep your information confidential. However, there are a few exceptions to the rule. If they suspect that you may seriously harm yourself or someone else, or in some court proceedings, they are obliged to report their suspicions. If, for instance, a health practitioner suspects that you have abused a child, they must contact the Children's Aid Society. If the client has a condition, including a mental health problem, that would make it dangerous for him or her to operate a motor vehicle, then a physician must report this to the Ministry of Transportation.

The courts can also subpoena your therapy records and your therapist's testimony under certain conditions, such as a sexual assault case. So it's a good idea to discuss with your therapist what he or she will include in your records, and how they will be kept.

Your therapist should explain confidentiality (privacy) issues with you at the beginning of the therapy.

NON-LICENSED THERAPISTS

Anyone can call themselves a psychotherapist and advertise their services, even if they don't have training. So it is important to find out what kind of experience the therapist has.

Non-licensed therapists do not belong to an organization that makes sure they're doing their job right. No one ensures that they are competent and ethical in their practices. And if clients have complaints, there is no one to handle them.

For more information about what to expect from your therapist, call his or her professional organization. This organization will have guidelines about supervision, training and ethics for its members. If you have a complaint about your therapist, call the governing or regulatory college to which he or she belongs.

QUESTION: Are therapists available in the evenings or on weekends?

ANSWER: Therapists can sometimes see clients in the morning before they go to work or at the end of the work day. However, it's often hard to get these time slots because many people want to see their therapists outside of regular office hours. It's unusual for a therapist to see clients on the weekend.

4

How much will therapy cost?

Psychotherapy from a psychiatrist or any other medical doctor is covered by OHIP, and will thus not cost you anything. Services obtained from other health care professionals (e.g., psychologists, social workers) may also be free if they are offered in government-funded hospitals, clinics or agencies. If psychotherapists work in a private practice, their services will not be covered by OHIP, and you will be charged a fee. These fees range from about $40 to $180 per hour. However, the fee will vary depending on the therapist's experience and training and the type of therapy. (Group therapy may be less expensive.) Some therapists offer a sliding scale, which means that they can offer a reduced fee based on your income.

Fees may also be covered through an extended health care plan or private insurance. (You may have a benefits plan through your work.) Some of these plans may only cover services up to a certain amount and for certain types of therapists (e.g., psychologists but not social workers).

If you are working in a large organization, you may have access to an employee assistance program (EAP)—sometimes referred to as an employee and family assistance program (EFAP). *(For more information about counselling services provided through EAPs and EFAPs, see Reducing job stress, p. 89, in Section 11.)*

If you are a student, counselling services will most likely be provided by your high school, college or university. Some communities also have free clinics, support groups and drop-in centres that offer counselling.

C̲S **CHALLENGE:** Many free services have long waiting lists.

SUGGESTIONS: Use a free service, such as a distress line, or go to a drop-in centre that has free groups. Get on several waiting lists at once. Tell them that if someone cancels, you can be available at the last minute. Keep checking in to find out where you are on the list. If you no longer need the services, ask them to remove your name from the list.

4

Types of therapy

Just like finding a therapist, choosing a type of therapy will be different for each person. It will depend on your problems, the approach you feel comfortable with and how long you want to be involved in therapy. Being a certain type of professional (e.g., social worker, psychiatrist) doesn't mean that the therapist will practise a certain type of therapy. In reality, many clinicians use a combination of different approaches.

Therapists' style will also vary. Some therapists will give you a lot of feedback about how they think you are doing and suggestions of what they think might help you. Other therapists will tend to be quieter during sessions, and will let you draw your own conclusions. You can tell therapists which approach you prefer, and ask them how they work. Therapists may be willing to adapt their style to suit your needs. If they can't, they may not be the right match for you.

2003 Centre for Addiction & Mental Health

QUESTION: How will I know if and when therapy is working?

ANSWER: Most likely when you start therapy, you'll have certain goals or ideas of what you'd like to be different. If you find that you are meeting these goals over time, chances are the therapy is making a difference. It's important to understand that results don't necessarily happen overnight. In fact, sometimes you'll feel worse at the start as issues are brought to the surface.

If you don't know if you are making progress in therapy, you should discuss this with your therapist. You may want to schedule times to evaluate how things are going in the sessions.

4

Studies indicate that only 15 per cent of successful therapies happen because of the model or technique a therapist uses. The most important factor for successful therapy is the quality of the relationship between the therapist and client.

Therapy can be short- or long-term. Because resources are often limited, you're more likely to receive short-term therapy, and then be linked to other service providers in the community.

BRIEF VS. LONG-TERM THERAPY

Brief therapy (e.g., solution-focused therapy), as its name implies, is a short-term therapy that often lasts between eight and 20 sessions. Short-term therapies are frequently used to deal with a specific problem, such as death, divorce, parenting issues or a specific phobia, rather than problems that have lasted for years. The sessions tend to focus more on current rather than childhood or other issues from the past. And the therapist generally takes an active role in guiding the discussions. Sometimes clients are given homework (e.g., exercises to help them cope with stress or anxiety between therapy sessions). Brief therapies are particularly helpful for depression and anxiety.

Long-term therapy (e.g., psychodynamic psychotherapy, psychoanalysis) is less structured than brief therapy. The client has more flexibility to talk about a variety of concerns related to both past and present issues. The length of therapy is indefinite, and can last a year or longer.

 QUESTION: How long will I need therapy?

ANSWER: How often you will need to go to therapy depends on the nature of your problems. You may have a concern that can be addressed in a few sessions. Or you may have more complicated issues that require about 20 sessions. Some people get therapy off and on throughout their lives.

4

MOST COMMON APPROACHES

Therapy can be quite different depending on the kind of approach being used. Therapy may focus on changing clients' behaviours or their way of thinking about the world. It can focus on understanding difficult situations from the past. Or it can focus on expressing feelings that have come from old wounds, such as a history of abuse. Therapy can also be about supporting a client through a difficult time. Four of the most common forms of psychotherapy now being practised are cognitive-behavioural therapy, interpersonal therapy, psychodynamic therapy and supportive therapy.

Cognitive-behavioural therapy is considered by many experts to be the number one way to treat depression and anxiety. It focuses on helping clients become aware of how certain negative automatic thoughts, attitudes, expectations and beliefs contribute to feelings of sadness and anxiety. Clients learn how these thinking patterns, which may have been developed in the past to deal with difficult or painful experiences, can be identified and changed in their day-to-day lives to reduce unhappiness. They learn to have more control over their moods by having more control over the way they think.

Interpersonal therapy focuses on identifying and resolving problems in establishing and maintaining satisfying relationships. These problems may include dealing with loss, life changes, couple difficulties or conflicts, and increasing the client's ease in social situations.

Psychodynamic therapy involves exploring the client's beliefs and inner states, even when the client may not be completely conscious of them. Psychodynamic therapy assumes that because clients may not be aware of what is causing their unhappiness, the usual methods for finding relief (e.g., talking to friends or family, getting advice) may not be helping. The therapy instead focuses on finding the underlying problems that show up in various ways (e.g., difficulties at work, problems in a relationship).

4

Supportive therapy involves providing support and advice during a difficult period. This form of therapy can be short- or long-term. It focuses more on current problems rather than long-term difficulties. The overall goal is to reduce clients' discomfort level and help them cope with their current circumstances.

INDIVIDUAL VS. COUPLE, FAMILY AND GROUP THERAPY

Whether you choose to see a therapist alone, with a partner, family member or as part of a group (with other participants you don't know) will depend on the kind of problem you want help with.

Family therapy is focused on changing the way families interact. It aims to increase understanding and improve communication among family members. It does so without placing blame on any one person. Family therapy is generally used when the family system is seen as contributing to one family member's difficulties (such as a child or adolescent's). Or it is used when one family member's difficulties are influencing other family members, and they need help in how to cope and adjust to the situation. Both the "identified client" (the person identified as having the problem) and the other family member(s) can benefit from this kind of therapy.

If you are looking for a family therapist, contact the Ontario Association for Marriage and Family Therapy at (416) 364-2627 in Toronto or toll-free at 1-800-267-2638. You can also view their Web site at www.oamft.on.ca.

Couple therapy helps couples to resolve problems and conflicts that they're unable to find solutions to on their own. Both partners sit down with the therapist and discuss their thoughts and feelings. This kind of therapy aims to help couples get to know themselves and each other better. If the couple wants to make changes, the therapist can help them do so.

If you are looking for a couple therapist, contact the Ontario Association for Marriage and Family Therapy at (416) 364-2627 in Toronto or toll-free at 1-800-267-2638. You can also view their Web site at www.oamft.on.ca.

Group therapy allows people to work on their problems by interacting with others in a group setting. Participants share their thoughts and feelings and receive feedback, encouragement and support from other members. This process enables them to learn more about how others respond to them. They can also practise new behaviours in the safety of the group. Group therapy can be particularly helpful for people dealing with relationship problems or difficulties with intimacy, self-esteem or trust. Some groups discuss issues as they're raised at the weekly sessions. Others stick to an agenda.

QUESTION: How long is each therapy session?

ANSWER: Individual sessions generally last between 20 to 50 minutes. Group sessions or family appointments can last longer.

2003 Centre for Addiction & Mental Health

QUESTION: How do I know I am getting the best treatment?

ANSWER: Good treatment is often based on a proper assessment. *(See Section 3: Getting an assessment, p. 21.)* It also involves following clear goals you have discussed and decided on with your therapist. To reach your treatment goals, you need a therapist who has education and experience with your kinds of issues, and is someone whom you can trust and respect.

4

Services at different life stages   5

Services for children and youth

Almost one in five children and youth has a mental health problem. These problems can show up in different ways. Children may be frequently sad or rebellious; have difficulty paying attention; have problems eating, sleeping or getting along with schoolmates; or they may skip school. As an adolescent, they may use alcohol or other drugs.

While it can be difficult to find mental health services for anyone, parents may find it particularly difficult to find services for children and youth. This is because these services fall under more government ministries, and involve more laws than adult services. There is also a shortage of child and adolescent mental health specialists, which can mean long waiting lists.

While it can be frustrating to find services for your child, don't give up! Try to be hopeful and be persistent. The Internet is a valuable tool for doing research. (*For a list of helpful Web sites and phone numbers, see Appendix B.*)

ASSESSMENT AND REFERRALS

Two-thirds of referrals to children's mental health services are for behavioural problems. Behavioural problems are more common among boys as boys are more likely to act out their problems. Girls, on the other hand, are more likely to hold in their problems, which can lead to emotional problems, such as depression and anxiety. Young people's difficulties often arise from stressful life events, such as abuse, neglect, a parent dying, parents divorcing or other major changes. Adolescents who struggle with gender identity and sexual orientation may develop feelings of loneliness and depression. Because of this, rates of suicide are higher among gay youth.

Children are unlikely to find mental health services on their own. They are usually referred by a family member, doctor, school, court or the Children's Aid Society. As teenagers, they may be able to refer themselves, but it depends on the agency's policies. At some agencies, therapists are required to tell the parents or caregivers that the youth has approached them.

Assessments can be done by many different specialists, including child or adolescent psychiatrists (who are specially trained to evaluate, diagnose and treat children and adolescents), nurses, child and youth workers, social workers or psychologists.

During an assessment, the specialist usually speaks to both the child and his or her parents, or any other adult who has referred the child. The specialist will ask each person's opinion of the child's problem. The specialist will also want to know, for example, how the child is doing at school and what the child's relationships are like with friends and family members. As well, the therapist will want to determine if the child has any medical problems that are affecting his or her mood, thoughts or behaviour. If the child is very young, the assessment may include other methods of evaluation. For instance, children may be asked to draw or play with certain toys if they can't use words to express themselves.

If the child is having emotional problems and learning difficulties, it is important to refer the child for academic or psychometric testing. This kind of testing assesses both the child's academic and emotional well-being. Psychometric testing can be provided by schools, hospitals or psychologists working in private practice. Because there are long waiting lists, parents may choose to have their child tested by private psychologists; however, this can be quite costly.

A child's assessment is rarely clear-cut. It can be difficult for parents to know if their adolescent's unusual behaviour or mood is a normal part of adolescent change or a real concern. Because of this, parents sometimes delay getting help. And before they know it, they have a crisis on their hands. Long waiting lists can prevent youth from getting help when the situation is critical.

Children's problems often come and go. They may seem to disappear for a while, and then return in a different form or during a stressful time. Because children are continually growing and changing, results of an assessment may suggest several different things that need to be done. These suggestions will depend on the child's stage of development and age. For instance, when the child is younger, the specialist may want to focus on language and speech or communication. As the child gets older, the specialist may suggest supportive therapy and possibly medication.

5

TREATMENT AND SUPPORT

Depending on the problem, a child could receive services from the following places:

- family doctor or general practitioner's office
- school (if a social worker or guidance counsellor is on site)
- youth clinic, mental health or addiction treatment centre or community residential treatment program
- children's mental health agency
- psychiatric unit of a children's hospital or psychiatric hospital
- private practice or
- program for young offenders, if the child or youth is in trouble with the law.

Children are usually treated in outpatient services. While they are rarely hospitalized, they may be if they:

- are a danger to themselves or others
- have been living in an unhealthy environment (e.g., an abusive home) or
- have experienced severe symptoms of an eating disorder or early onset depression, schizophrenia or bipolar disorder.

Various specialists may be involved in a child's care (e.g., psychologists, child and youth workers, nurses, child and adolescent psychiatrists, speech or language therapists and families). Children benefit from the many perspectives provided by a team of professionals.

5

Treatment for children or youth generally consists of:

- working with parents to teach them ways to avoid conflict and to be supportive when interacting with their child. This is an increasingly common part of treatment that may include educational or parents' groups.
- psychotherapy, with the child individually and with participating family members. *(For more information on family therapy, see p. 39 in Section 4.)* The therapist may use a cognitive-behavioural approach *(see p. 38 in Section 4 for a definition)* or offer supportive counselling. Because there are often many people involved in a child's care, a case manager may also help co-ordinate services provided by the various caregivers. These caregivers work in schools, hospitals or the community.
- medication. However, medication is prescribed less often to children than adults. Parents' and professionals' first choice for treatment isn't usually medication. This is because there is little, if any, research on the long-term effects on growing children. Yet research shows that therapies that work to change behaviour do work, so these are often preferred.

Parents and professionals have to consider the potential benefits of medication for the child. Will using the medication mean the child will lead a happier life? Will the child have an easier time growing up? Will there be less disruption in the child's development? Parents and professionals also have to consider the potential side-effects of the medication. Parents should be aware that schools may encourage medication as a way to manage or control a child's behaviour. If a doctor or teacher recommends medication for your child, it is important to determine if he or she is simply harder to handle or is affected by a mental health problem. *(For more information on medication, see Taking medication, p. 55, in Section 7.)*

Services for older adults

The percentage of adults 55 years of age and over is growing. As we age, our needs change. Our need for health care, social services and institutional care tends to increase. And yet the needs of older adults are often neglected.

The main mental health problems affecting older adults are dementias (along with paranoia), depression and anxiety. They may also experience many other problems, including physical health problems, grief over friends or partners dying, feelings of isolation and loneliness, language barriers, stress around recent immigration and abuse.

Older adults are most commonly abused financially (e.g., by theft or fraud). However, the abuse may also be physical. For example, an adult child may hit, slap or punch an older adult. Or the abuse may be psychological (e.g., when partners or adult children are critical, controlling or threatening).

Older adults tend to be referred to mental health specialists by other adults (e.g., a family member or caretaker.) These people often have the difficult task of figuring out if the older adult's behaviour or mood is normal. Is their behaviour just a part of growing old, or is it something to be concerned about? For instance, memory or concentration problems may be a result of the aging process. Or these problems could be related to dementias, depression or other mental health problems. Problems such as misuse or overuse of alcohol and prescription drugs may be difficult to detect and can affect the older adult's abilities. Older adults often have to rely on others to refer them for services. This means they may not get services until their situation has reached a crisis and someone else decides it is time for them to seek help.

The shame and stigma associated with mental health problems can be particularly severe for older adults. They grew up in a time when there was less openness and understanding of mental health problems. Unfortunately, the fear of being discriminated against, along with the fear of being put in a hospital, often prevent older adults from seeking help on their own.

5

ASSESSMENT AND REFERRALS

Older adults are usually assessed by a family doctor or geriatric outreach team. These teams are made up of doctors, social workers, nurses and occupational therapists. The assessment generally takes place in the older adult's home to see how the person manages and to find out if changes are needed to make it easier and safer to continue living at home. To see a geriatric psychiatry team, older adults usually require a referral from their family doctor.

TREATMENT AND SUPPORT

While older adults usually receive care from geriatric psychiatrists or geriatric outreach teams, in general, there are not enough professionals to respond adequately to their needs. Treatment usually consists of support, education for family and caregivers, and possibly medication. Team members work with community agencies to provide the support needed.

Treatment for older adults may also include addiction services.

Other care for older adults with mental health problems tends to be mainly social services, rather than actual treatment for mental health problems. These social services may be offered through:

- seniors' clubs
- drop-in centres
- Meals on Wheels, which delivers meals to the home and
- Community Care Access Centres (CCAC). *(See Home care, p. 68, in Section 8.)* CCACs mainly provide in-home support services (e.g., a personal support worker comes to the home to prepare meals for older adults who need help with activities of daily living).

5

Natural healing

6

Many people choose to use natural therapies to help them cope with a mental health problem. These therapies can be less intrusive than medical treatments. They tend to focus more on preventing illness, and promoting self-healing and healthy living. Natural practitioners generally focus more than medical practitioners on the client's overall well-being (mind, body *and* spirit). They also tend to spend more time with clients than medical practitioners.

These therapies are often used in addition to other more traditional approaches. However, some people find that treatments such as acupuncture, naturopathic remedies or meditation are enough to help them reduce stress and get through difficult times. Still other people may choose traditional healing practices used by the culture or group within which they have lived.

Body work

Many therapies involve working with the body to influence the mind. Many of these approaches to healing, such as biofeedback, acupuncture, reflexology, reiki and shiatsu, are drawn from ancient Eastern-based practices. They work to realign the body's energy; reduce stress, anxiety and physical pain; and increase feelings of relaxation.

Shiatsu is a Japanese massage treatment that involves applying physical pressure (through the thumbs, knees and elbows) along energy paths called meridians. Shiatsu treatments help balance or regulate the body's energy, which is influenced by stress, fatigue, muscle tension and other health problems.

Biofeedback is a technique in which people are taught to use signals from their own bodies to give them feedback about their health.

Acupuncture uses similar principles of healing as shiatsu. But instead of applying manual pressure, the practitioner inserts needles into specific points on the skin to regulate the body's flow of energy.

These practices are not covered by OHIP, and are generally not covered by extended health care plans. An exception is Swedish massage. This may be covered by an extended health care plan for up to a certain amount each year if done by a registered massage therapist. Shiatsu is occasionally covered by extended health care benefits.

> To get a referral to a Swedish massage therapist in your area, contact the Ontario Massage Therapist Association at (416) 979-2010 in Toronto, or call toll-free at 1-800-668-2022. To find an acupuncturist, contact the Ontario Association of Acupuncture and Traditional Chinese Medicine at (416) 944-2265 in Toronto. To find a shiatsu therapist, call the Shiatsu Therapy Association of Ontario at (416) 923-7826 in Toronto or toll-free at 1-877-923-7826. For information about biofeedback, view the Web site for the Association for Applied Psychophysiology and Biofeedback in the United States at www.aapb.org.

Creative therapies

Creative activities, such as art, music, writing, photography, drama, drawing and play, give people a way to explore their feelings and thoughts. These activities also allow people to express themselves in an artistic manner. Creative therapies help clients express and unravel their inner conflicts. They are often available in hospitals, treatment facilities, private practices and in community programs and art therapy schools.

Nutrition and naturopathy

Having a balanced diet is a good way to take care of yourself. It is also key to maintaining your mental health. You may choose to supplement your diet with vitamins and minerals or herbal remedies.

Like traditional medications, "natural" therapies can also have side-effects. Herbal therapies may interact with prescription drugs and affect other health conditions. If you use these kinds of remedies, make sure to tell your doctor.

Clinical dietitians will work with you to identify nutritional problems. They will also assess and monitor changes to your diet. Registered dietitians are health professionals with a university degree in food and nutrition. They have at least one year's practical experience.

Naturopathic doctors are health care professionals trained to use natural methods to promote healing. The therapies they may use include homeopathy, clinical nutrition, traditional Chinese medicine, and botanical or herbal medicine. They have at least three years of premedical training and four years at an accredited college. Most extended health care insurance plans cover naturopathy up to a certain amount each year.

6

> To get a referral to a nutritional professional, call Dietitians of Canada at (416) 596-0857 in Toronto, or view their Web site at www.dietitians.ca. The College of Dietitians of Ontario can be reached at (416) 598-1725 in Toronto or toll-free at 1-800-668-4990. Or view their Web site at www.cdo.on.ca.

> To get a referral to a naturopathic doctor, call the Ontario Association of Naturopathic Doctors' referral line at (416) 233-2001 ext. 24 in Toronto or toll-free at 1-877-628-7284. Or view their Web site at www.oand.org.

Spiritual healing

There is growing evidence connecting religion and spirituality to overall health and well-being. This includes prevention and recovery from various mental health problems.

Praying and regularly going to religious or worship services may reduce stress, help promote calm and help people to be more outwardly focused. As a result, people can recover faster, have less serious side-effects, be hospitalized less and feel less anxious and depressed.

There are many other forms of religious and spiritual practice. People can benefit from practices such as Aboriginal healing circles, sweat lodges and ceremonies, Shamanistic rituals, Zen meditation and Hindu-based yoga and breathing exercises

Spirituality can also be expressed through art, nature, music and writing.

You can find out about yoga classes by looking up "yoga" in the Yellow Pages of your phone book. Or call a local health club or community centre to see if they offer classes. Meditation is sometimes offered through a yoga or a spiritual centre, and generally costs about the same as yoga, or less. Once you've learned these techniques, you can do them at home.

CHALLENGE: Natural therapies generally aren't covered by health insurance plans and can be very expensive.

SUGGESTIONS: There are many ways you can help your body heal naturally without spending lots of money. Here are some ideas:

- Take a bath with Epsom salts to relax.
- Learn how to massage your own hands and feet, or—better yet—get your partner or a friend to give you a massage.
- Drink herbal tea.
- Go for a bike ride or take a long walk. Endurance exercises can help release endorphins in the brain that reduce depression and lift your spirits.
- Lift weights or stretch.
- Get a yoga tape so that you can do yoga at home.

Medical services

7

Taking medication

There tend to be strong and conflicting views on taking medication. Many people are happy to find a pill that decreases their suffering and improves their quality of life. Others do not find medication helpful at all. They may be disturbed by side-effects that are unpleasant and even debilitating or unknown in the long-term. And they may not like the idea that the drug alters the way they think and feel. Some may view their need to take medication as a sign of weakness. Still others may be concerned about addiction. Or they may be discouraged because the drug isn't as effective as they had hoped.

Even those people who find that medication is useful may still experience side-effects that make it difficult for them to continue to take their prescriptions. Many people have to try two or more medications before they find one that they can tolerate (e.g., has few or no side-effects) and which is effective. This is because it is often difficult to predict which drug will work best for which person.

It is up to you to decide whether medication is right for you. Should you decide to take medication, your body may have to adjust to it before your doctor can assess how long you'll need to take it and the amount of the dose. The doctor's opinion may change, depending on how your body reacts to or absorbs the drug and as new research evolves.

A doctor may gradually increase the dose to figure out the amount needed to get the best effect from a drug. The drug will most likely come in a pill or tablet form. Liquids or injections (short- or long-acting) may be recommended for treating certain kinds of conditions.

Establish a relationship with one pharmacist you trust, particularly when you are taking several different medications. This way, the pharmacist will be aware of all the medications you've been prescribed and will be able to tell you about possible interactions. But don't rely just on your pharmacist for information: speak to other experts and read up on the medications.

QUESTION: What if the medication doesn't work?

ANSWER: Not every medication works for every person. Unfortunately, doctors can't always predict which medication will work for you. But it's easier for them to choose the right drug if they have some details. Which medications have worked for you or a close relative in the past? What are your symptoms? What other medications are you taking?

Ask your health care provider when you'll see results from the medication. Some anti-anxiety medications can work within 30 minutes. Antidepressants can take from four to six weeks to become fully effective. Some antipsychotics can take even longer to help all symptoms. While it can be extremely frustrating to wait, you will have to give it some time. Find other ways to get support and care in the meantime.

If your medication is not working, your doctor can adjust the dose, prescribe another medication to complement the first or switch you to a different medication. Researchers are studying a number of new medications and treatments, which may be available in the future.

Remember that medication is only one tool to help treat mental health problems. You can also take medication in combination with psychotherapy, joining a support group, talking to friends and family or eating a well-balanced diet.

TYPES OF MEDICATION

There are various types of psychiatric drugs:

Anti-anxiety medications, previously known as anxiolytics or minor tranquilizers, are used to help calm people and relieve anxiety. Commonly used anti-anxiety medications are diazepam (Valium®) and lorazepam (Ativan®).

Antidepressants are most commonly used to treat depression. They are also used to treat different forms of anxiety, severe premenstrual mood changes and bulimia. Commonly used antidepressants include fluoxetine (Prozac®), sertraline (Zoloft®) and venlafaxine (Effexor®).

Antipsychotics, also called neuroleptics, are used to treat symptoms of acute or chronic psychosis, including schizophrenia, mania and organic disorders. Some of the most common antipsychotics are risperidone (Risperdal®), olanzapine (Zyprexa®), haloperidol (Haldol®) and clozapine (Clozaril®).

7

Mood stabilizers are used to help control mood swings (extreme highs and lows) connected with bipolar disorder and prevent further episodes of this condition. Commonly used mood stabilizers are lithium (Lithane®, Duralith®) and divalproex (Epival®).

Please note that while some of the more common drugs are listed above, this does not imply that CAMH endorses the use of these particular medications over others.

SIDE-EFFECTS

Side-effects can be minor or serious, and vary greatly from person to person. Common side-effects include:

• minor stomach problems (nausea, constipation, diarrhea)
• sexual difficulties
• dizziness
• dry mouth
• blurred vision

- allergic reactions
- fatigue or difficulty getting to sleep
- twitching and trembling
- akathisia (restlessness, feeling like you have to move your legs, especially at night) and
- weight gain.

A particularly serious side-effect that can be caused by antipsychotics is tardive dyskinesia. This is an involuntary movement, usually of the tongue, lips, jaw or fingers, that can be permanent.

Which side-effects you experience depend on the drug and dose you are taking and how sensitive you are to the medication. In most cases, side-effects lessen as therapy continues. But it is also true that side-effects may not develop immediately. If you did not have certain symptoms before taking the medication, it's possible that they are a result of the medication.

7

If you do experience side-effects, do not stop or change your medication without first talking to your doctor, pharmacist, nurse or caseworker to find out how to cope with them. If the doctor dismisses your concerns, persist with your questions. Then consider getting a referral to someone else if you are not satisfied with the care you are receiving.

If the doctor's suggestions don't work, he or she can:

- prescribe another drug to counteract the unpleasant effects of the drug
- switch you to a different drug
- reduce the dose of the drug or
- gradually withdraw you from the drug.

Your doctor should continually monitor your medication. In some cases, he or she will test your blood to make sure your liver and other organs are functioning well and that the drug levels in your bloodstream are okay.

To find out about the effects of prescription and over-the-counter drugs as well as herbal products during pregnancy or while breastfeeding, call the Motherisk information line at (416) 813-6780 in Toronto. For information about the effects of alcohol, nicotine and drugs such as marijuana, cocaine and ecstasy during pregnancy or while breastfeeding, call Motherisk's toll-free Alcohol and Substance Use Helpline at 1-877-327-4636. Their Web site is www.motherisk.org.

For health-related questions, call Telehealth Ontario, a free 24-hour confidential information line. Registered nurses, with support from pharmacists, will respond to your concerns. Their toll-free number is 1-866-797-0000 and TTY is 1-800-387-5559. Their Web site is www.gov.on.ca/health/english/program/telehealth/telehealth_mn.html.

QUESTION: I have heard that psychiatric medications have bad side-effects. Is this true?

ANSWER: Most side-effects from psychiatric medications are mild and temporary. However, some have serious, long-term effects that you should know about. Tell your health care providers about any side-effects. Don't worry about bothering them. If you don't tell them you are having a problem, they can't help you solve it. Ask family members to help. Explain the signs of a serious side-effect, so they can watch for them. It is also important to discuss the risks and benefits of taking or not taking the medication with your doctor.

If you have questions about your medication, bring them up with your health care providers. It's a good idea to write down questions so you will remember to ask them at your next appointment.

Your doctor, pharmacist or other health care provider can help you deal with these side-effects. For instance, if a drug makes you drowsy, they may suggest that you take it at night. If a drug nauseates you, they may recommend that you take it with food.

7

MIXING MEDICATION WITH OTHER SUBSTANCES

Tell your doctor or pharmacist about any over-the-counter medication, vitamins, herbal products, illegal drugs or homeopathic remedies that you are taking. This is important because they may interact with the prescription drug. Ask about caffeine, alcohol and grapefruit juice, too. Grapefruit juice does not interact with all medications, but can cause serious side-effects and even be toxic with some.

GOING OFF MEDICATION

If you want to go off your medication, first consult with your doctor. If you suddenly stop taking your medication, you could experience withdrawal symptoms or the return of the symptoms you were originally being treated for (e.g., insomnia after stopping to take a sleeping pill). You may also experience other symptoms, such as nausea, headaches and dizziness.

7

Withdrawal symptoms usually start within hours or a day or two of stopping a medication. Sometimes even missing two consecutive doses can cause withdrawal. Recurrence or return of the original problems can occur within a few days, but can also happen weeks or months later. It can sometimes be difficult to tell the difference between withdrawal and recurrence of the original problem.

If you decide with your doctor to go off your medication or switch to another drug, your current dose will be tapered. This means that the amount of medication you are taking will be slowly reduced. This happens over a few days to several weeks, decreasing your chances of withdrawal. The severity of withdrawal symptoms you may experience depends on the type of medication you've been taking, how long you've been taking it and your dose.

QUESTION: Will I have to be on medication for the rest of my life?

ANSWER: Not necessarily. The length of time you will stay on a medication depends on many different factors:

- the type of mental health problem
- what symptoms you have and how long you've had them
- how many relapses (recurrence of the symptoms) you have experienced
- how severe your symptoms have been and
- what other supports you have in your life.

Some people can be treated for a mental health problem over a short period, and recover fully. However, some problems are longer term and require indefinite treatment. Certain medications, such as sleeping pills and anti-anxiety medication, should be used for only a short time while you are learning new techniques and skills for coping.

For a first episode of depression, antidepressants should be taken for about one year. Antidepressants can be taken longer or indefinitely if you have more than two relapses or the symptoms in your first episode were very serious. Mood stabilizers and antipsychotics are usually taken indefinitely, because both bipolar disorder and schizophrenia, for which they are pre-scribed, are long-term problems.

Talk to your doctor about how long you will need to take the medication. Ask about how effective the medication is compared to psychotherapy. You may also want to discuss your feelings about taking medication. The most common mistake people make is stopping their medication when they feel better. While some medications are intended to treat only serious conditions, most psychiatric medications are meant to prevent further relapses. It is possible that your dose of medication can be lowered, or that you can gradually go off the medication, but be sure to speak to your doctor first. In many instances, a combination of medication and therapy is the most effective approach.

7

QUESTIONS TO ASK ABOUT MEDICATION

What are the generic and trade names of my medication?

What dose should I take?

Why am I taking this medication and what is it supposed to do?

How and when do I take this medication? (e.g., Do I need to take it at the same time each day, with food?)

What are the most common side-effects, and how can they be treated?

What are the signs of a more serious drug reaction that I should contact my doctor about?

Which drugs, food and alcohol interact with this medication?

What should I do if I miss a dose?

How long will I be taking this medication?

When can I expect the drug to start working?

Can I get addicted to the medication?

What research is there about the drug I'm being prescribed (e.g., its effectiveness, risks, recommended dose)?

What would be involved in going off the medication?

What are the long-term effects of being on the medication?

QUESTION: Is this medication addictive?

ANSWER: Most psychiatric medications are not addictive. Many are intended to be taken for a long time or indefinitely, but that does not mean they are addictive. Mental health problems involve a chemical imbalance, and just like other non-psychiatric problems, they often need long-term treatment.

Some psychiatric medications, such as anti-anxiety medications and stimulants used to treat attention-deficit/hyperactivity disorder, can become addictive, even when they are taken as prescribed. If you have any concerns about this, don't hesitate to speak to your doctor, pharmacist or health care provider. Tell your doctor if you know you have problems with addiction, so the doctor can be careful about the types of medication he or she prescribes.

Electroconvulsive therapy

Electroconvulsive therapy (ECT) is most commonly used for people who have severe depression for whom other treatments have not worked. ECT can be very effective for these people; however, it remains highly controversial.

The client is given an anaesthetic and a muscle relaxant. Then an electric charge is applied to the brain that induces a small seizure. Almost all people who are treated with ECT experience some memory loss of what happened immediately before or during the treatment. In some cases, clients lose the memory of significant periods in their lives.

Like other treatments for mental health problems, it is important to get all the facts about ECT and its potential side-effects before you decide whether this treatment is right for you.

More intensive and specialized support   8

There are various forms of specialized care for people with severe and continuing mental health problems who have many complex needs.

Assertive community treatment (ACT) teams

Assertive community treatment (ACT) teams may include a psychiatrist, psychologist, psychiatric nurse, social worker, peer support worker (someone with a similar problem or issue who offers support), caseworker, recreation therapist, addiction specialist, vocational (job) specialist and/or occupational therapist who help you with tasks for day-to-day living. Teams often have up to 10 members. Some of the team members are linked to a hospital. Others are based in the community and may work with a local hospital close to where the client lives.

ACT teams offer intensive case management and support for people with severe and continuing mental health problems (e.g., people who may have been hospitalized often, and who need help taking medication or following a prescription, finding a place to live or using work and other support services). ACT team members often meet with the client every day in the person's community (e.g., in the person's home or in a coffee shop). They provide services on a long-term basis to make sure people receive consistent care and strong, ongoing support from the same group of health care workers.

Most of the time, you can get ACT team services through a mental health agency. Like many other services, you may be more likely to find ACT teams in cities and larger communities.

Intensive case management

Intensive case management is similar to the support offered by ACT teams. The difference is that it tends to be provided by nurses or social workers working one-on-one with the person, rather than as part of a team. Case managers see their clients regularly to co-ordinate the person's care and services. They can provide more one-on-one support than outpatient services, for example.

Specialized outpatient services in psychiatric facilities

Specialized outpatient services include special intensive programs, rehabilitation for people with severe and chronic (long-term) problems, and community support through case managers. Specialized services may also include day programs. Clients may participate in educational groups or receive help with medication, which may be checked and given out as part of the day program.

8

CHALLENGE: Many mental health workers do not have specialized training to respond to certain kinds of problems or needs. Some examples where special training may be helpful include treating people with more than one problem, such as:

• a mental health and an addiction problem or concurrent disorder
• a mental health problem and a developmental disability or dual diagnosis or
• a mental health problem and physical disability.

Health care workers may also need training to help people from different communities: for example, children or older adults; people from specific ethnoracial/ethnocultural groups; people who are lesbian, bisexual, gay, transgendered or transsexual; or people whose needs are not satisfied by existing programs (like someone who can't live completely independently but does not need to be in a group home).

SUGGESTIONS: Generally, you have two main options if you are looking for specialized services. You can go to hospitals and health care agencies or you can contact an organization that serves your particular community (e.g., an organization that focuses on helping immigrants and refugees or people with a dual diagnosis).

Specialized services are not very common, so you are more likely to get services from an agency serving the general population. Even if someone does not have specialized training, that person will often have experience working with people from diverse cultures and backgrounds. If you look for mental health services from this type of agency, you may want to ask if they offer the kind of clinic, program or expertise that meets your particular needs (e.g., a cultural interpreter, a concurrent disorder program for people with both a mental health and addiction problem, or a youth clinic for a teenager). If you contact a community organization, they may be able to offer informal counselling, or link or refer you to a mental health agency.

8

Forensic services

People with mental health problems who break the law (forensic clients) may be placed in forensic psychiatric facilities or community programs, with certain conditions.

People who have committed non-violent or low risk offences (e.g., mischief, minor theft) may be able to enter diversion programs. Diversion programs are set up by the courts as a way to redirect clients and connect them to mental health treatment services or supports. They prevent some people from going to jail and having a criminal record.

You can refer yourself to a diversion program or be referred by a family member, friend or defence lawyer (or duty counsel, if you don't have a lawyer). Court support workers are located in many courts to help you deal with the court system. They help make sure that your case goes through the courts and that alternative sentencing is considered. They can also help you get into supportive housing.

8

Forensic clients can also use assertive community treatment (ACT) programs, community supports and other mental health services in the community or receive specialized services in certain hospitals.

> To find out more about diversion programs, contact a local community mental health agency, or call Legal Aid Ontario at (416) 979-1446 in Toronto or toll-free at 1-800-668-8258.

Home care

Case managers, community support workers, social workers, psychiatric nurses, occupational therapists and other health care workers can visit you at home to provide help with daily living (e.g., shopping for groceries, preparing a budget). They can help support your family and friends, while helping you make the best use of your own strengths. Assertive community treatment (ACT) team members may also conduct home visits. *(See Assertive community treatment (ACT) teams, p. 65.)*

COMMUNITY CARE ACCESS CENTRES (CCACS)

Community care access centres are one type of community agency that provides home care. There are 43 CCACs across the province that offer health and personal support services, including home care for people who are less mobile. First, CCAC case managers assess the types of services and amount of help the client needs. Depending on the client's needs, they can provide nursing, social work, occupational therapy, physiotherapy, nutrition counselling, help with daily living (such as bathing and cleanliness or getting dressed) and other care.

Anyone can make a referral to CCAC services, including family members, friends, caregivers, health care professionals—and clients themselves. However, CCAC services vary within communities across the province. Where CCAC services are limited or unavailable, you may have to find other forms of support.

> To find the phone number of the CCAC nearest you, contact the Ministry of Health and Long-Term Care at (416) 314-5518 in Toronto or toll-free at 1-800-268-1154.

CHALLENGE: For programs that don't offer in-home visits, transportation can be a problem. This is particularly true for people living in isolated areas, rural communities, small towns or on First Nations reserves; and for people with physical or developmental disabilities, people whose first language is not English and people with low incomes.

SUGGESTIONS: Sometimes in-home care is available. In a crisis, contact a 24-hour distress line. (These phone numbers are listed at the front of your phone book.) Or call the police at 911 if you fear danger to yourself or others.

If you are receiving ODSP (Ontario Disability Support Program) benefits, check to see if the benefits include transportation costs for medical appointments or job training. You can also look into Internet support groups.

In an emergency or crisis

9

What is an emergency or crisis?

A crisis is a time of danger or great difficulty. Generally, you will know you are in crisis if you feel like you can't cope and are not in control. For instance, you may be having difficulty sleeping, eating, paying attention or carrying on your normal routine at home, work or school. Or you may have had a serious setback or be wondering if you can keep going. Acting on thoughts of suicide—for example, cutting your wrists—is an emergency.

A crisis could result from losing your housing, problems with money, worries about your child's well-being, or a problem or difficult situation that is not cleared up and becomes more serious over time. What is a difficult situation for one person may be a crisis for another, depending on the person's support system, and how he or she interprets and copes with the problem.

Some people show no signs when they are in crisis. In other people, it is obvious when they are having a hard time. They may behave differently and may not think clearly.

SUICIDE

Some people may have thoughts of suicide or have even made suicide attempts. They may feel so hopeless and despairing about their lives that they see dying as the only way out of their difficulties.

More women attempt suicide than men. But more men actually die as a result of suicide because the methods men use are more likely to cause death. Suicide also tends to be more common among people with serious depression, bipolar disorder (formerly called manic depression), schizophrenia; people with substance use problems; people with few social supports; Inuit living in the North; and youth who are lesbian, gay, bisexual, transsexual or transgendered who may be struggling with gender identity issues, and experiencing prejudice and discrimination.

Crisis intervention—stepping in to help a person in crisis—involves providing treatment and support as soon as possible after you know the person is in distress. *(For information on preparing a crisis plan and having someone admitted to a hospital, see Take action, p. 110, in Section 12.)*

In an emergency, call 911.

Types of crisis services

Here are some ways to get help in a crisis.

EMERGENCY DEPERTMENTS OF HOSPITALS

You can go to the emergency department of a hospital for help. However, unless you are a danger to yourself or others, the health care professional (e.g., doctor, nurse) at the hospital may suggest you return home or stay with a friend or family member as long as you have someone with you for support.

Choosing to be admitted to the hospital is a personal decision. Some people find it stressful to be in a hospital where they are separated from their usual supports and must follow rules and regulations and structured programs. *(For more information about getting an assessment in emergency departments of hospitals, see p. 24 in Section 3.)*

QUESTION: When is it necessary for someone to be hospitalized?

ANSWER: Hospitalization is usually only recommended when outpatient services cannot adequately meet the care needs of a person's condition or the person's challenges of daily living.

You may prefer to be in the hospital, surrounded by a support system and away from your day-to-day responsibilities where your need for medication can be assessed—or if you are already using medication, you can be observed for possible side-effects.

However, if you have supports in the community, it may be better for you not to be in the hospital as long as you feel safe. Being in the hospital can be very disruptive to your life; for example, it may be difficult to keep up social contacts or deal with financial or housing issues. However, you can be forced into hospital in certain situations. *(See Appendix C.)*

Outpatients have a variety of programs available to them. Having regular, pre-set appointments are often helpful during a difficult time.

QUESTION: If I am hospitalized, how long will it last?

ANSWER: With fewer hospital beds available across the province and greater efforts to offer supports within the community, generally people are only hospitalized for serious problems and for a short time. Usually, hospital stays are for two weeks or less.

9

MOBILE CRISIS UNITS AND SERVICES

A mobile crisis unit can provide help in a crisis over the phone or at a person's home. A worker will assess the situation, help to lessen the present crisis and decide on the best way to deal with the problem. Both new and existing clients receive a psychiatric consultation if needed. They are assessed and treated on the spot and connected with other useful services.

Like many other health care services, mobile crisis units are more likely to be found in cities and larger communities. However, a greater number of these units are now operating, with some variations, to provide more service to rural areas.

To reach a mobile crisis unit, call 911, or contact your local hospital, community mental health agency or a community care access centre.

DISTRESS AND CRISIS LINES

Distress or crisis phone lines are open 24 hours a day if you need to talk to someone. Crisis hotlines offer free, anonymous telephone counselling and information. The counsellors must keep everything you say confidential. Trained volunteers usually run these phone support services.

There are different types of hotlines; for example, assaulted women or rape crisis hotlines, suicide lines and kids' help lines. Distress lines outside of cities are a major source of support and can link you to local services.

You can find emergency numbers at the front of your phone book or through a local community information centre. For the phone number of a community information centre or distress line near you, call 211 in Toronto or (416) 397-4636 if you are outside of Toronto. (For a list of hotlines, see Appendix A.)

9

SAFE HOUSES AND SHELTERS

Shelters offer a safe, temporary place to live during a crisis where workers can give you advice and support. Shelters and safe houses often provide services to specific groups of people; for example, women only, women and children, men only or youth. They may offer housing services, counselling and other supports along with providing a bed and a meal. *(See Housing, p. 99, in Section 11.)*

Note: Some shelters or safe houses have policies that exclude people with mental health or substance use problems.

For a list of shelters in your area for women who have been abused, view the Web site www.shelternet.ca.

For information on distress centres in Ontario, view the Web site www.dcontario.org. For Ontario crisis centres, refer to http://crisis.vianet.on.ca.

FOOD AND SHELTER

The Out of the Cold program was started up in Toronto more than 15 years ago to help provide shelter, food and warm clothing for people without homes and people with low incomes. The program provides people with meals and shelter during the colder months and, in some cases, year-round. Toronto has about 40 Out of the Cold overnight programs and more than 20 meal programs. The program also runs in about seven other Ontario cities.

Food banks, community kitchens and other food services are also available in some communities for people who need them.

To find the location of an Out of the Cold program in Toronto, call (416) 782-0122 or view their Web site at www.ootcrc.com.

9

Community
supports

10

Community supports could mean anything from self-help groups (where people with similar problems help and support each other) to support from community workers to distress lines. Here is a more detailed look at some community supports. *(For more information, see Section 8: More intensive and specialized support, p. 65.)*

Consumer/survivor initiatives

People who have a mental health problem or people who have used mental health services or programs sometimes describe themselves as consumer/survivors. (Some people believe they "survived" a mental health problem. Others see themselves as having survived the mental health system—depending on their experiences.)

Consumer/survivor initiatives are run by and for people who use or have used the mental health system. They were created as an alternative to traditional mental health services. These programs offer education, information and support from people who have had similar experiences. They also provide social and recreational activities, work opportunities and employment in an alternative business.

These programs may be able to help you start up your own business, learn more about a mental health issue that affects you or do work as an advocate. An advocate is someone who fights for a cause, such as better services for a particular group of people with a specific mental health problem.

The Ontario Peer Development Initiative (OPDI) offers support and training to consumer/survivor groups and organizations in Ontario. These consumer/survivor initiatives may involve working in areas such as self-help and peer support, business start-up and growth, knowledge production and skills training, advocacy, public education, professional education, and artistic and cultural activities.

> To get the name and phone number of a consumer/survivor program (e.g., self-help group, consumer business, self-advocacy program) near you, contact the OPDI, formerly called the Consumer/Survivor Development Initiative, at (416) 484-8785 in Toronto or toll-free at 1-866-681-6661. Or view their Web site at www.opdi.org.

> To get work experience, contact the Ontario Council of Alternative Businesses (OCAB). *(For more information on OCAB, see Types of work, p. 88, in Section 11.)*

Community mental health services

Mental health services in the community can be offered through mental health agencies, clubhouses, drop-in centres or outpatient community health clinics.

MENTAL HEALTH AGENCIES

10

The Canadian Mental Health Association (CMHA) is one of the largest mental health organizations in the province. Its Ontario division has 33 regional agencies across the province. These local CMHA branches are a good place to start to find out what services and resources there are in your community.

CMHA offices will refer you to other mental health centres in your area. They also offer counselling, case management, housing, clubhouses, grief support groups, information and assertive community treatment (ACT) teams. They can help co-ordinate your care and provide day-to-day support.

To find the CMHA agency nearest you, call the Ontario division's main office at (416) 977-5580 in Toronto or toll-free at 1-800-875-6213. Or view their Web site at www.ontario.cmha.ca.

Contact the community information centre in your neighbourhood to find supports and services near you.

CLUBHOUSES

Clubhouses are a place where people with serious mental health problems can go for a sense of belonging and community. Members socialize, develop skills and work side-by-side with staff in the daily operation of the clubhouse. They may prepare meals, do office or maintenance work or other jobs. Some clubhouses also offer transitional employment or housing support programs.

Clubhouses differ from other mental health services in that consumer/survivors, in partnership with staff, run the clubhouse, rather than simply receiving services.

Clubhouses can be accessed through the Ontario Peer Development Initiative (OPDI), your local CMHA office or other mental health service providers. Progress Place, the first clubhouse in Canada and the largest, lists other Ontario clubhouses on its Web site at www.progressplace.org.

10

DROP-IN CENTRES

Drop-in centres focus more on providing recreational and social opportunities than work experience. They may have organized programs; for example, craft classes, recreational activities, meals and educational sessions. Or people may use the centre to drop by for a coffee, have a rest, play a board game, meet with friends, use the phone or computer or, in some facilities, take a shower or do laundry. Some drop-in centres also provide counselling.

Self-help groups

Self-help, or mutual aid, groups are made up of people who share a common issue or mental health problem (e.g., abuse, grief, addiction, depression) in themselves or a family member. These groups are usually open-ended, so you can join in or leave the group at any time. Consumer/ survivors or their family members who have experience in the mental health system usually lead the groups. Many people find it rewarding to volunteer in these organizations and share what they have learned with others.

Group members generally gather in informal meetings where they give and receive support and exchange information and ideas on coping and solving problems. The main goal is to decrease feelings of isolation by sharing their experiences with people who will understand what they're going through. Self-help meetings are free, anonymous and confidential.

You can also find self-help groups on the Internet. You can join an on-line support group to offer and receive support, discuss issues and problems, and share information. There is more secrecy since you don't meet face-to-face with the group. And you don't have to travel, so people living in remote areas or people with physical disabilities can easily take part. However, you should be careful. You cannot be sure that information you receive on the Internet is accurate or that everyone you communicate with will be responsible and honest.

10

Find out about self-help organizations through your local mental health association, community mental health services, family doctor or adver-tisements or listings in newspapers. Also, the larger Toronto branches of provincial organizations sometimes offer expanded mental health services (e.g., lectures and groups) for people both in Toronto and outside the city, if you can travel.

To join a self-help group on depression or bipolar disorder, call the Mood Disorders Association of Ontario at (416) 486-8046 in Toronto or toll-free at 1-888-486-8236. To join a self-help group on schizophrenia, call the Schizophrenia Society of Ontario at (416) 449-6830 in Toronto or toll-free at 1-800-449-6367.

To start your own self-help group, solve a group problem or help someone to help themselves, contact the Ontario Self-Help Network (OSHNET) at (416) 487-4355 in Toronto or toll-free at 1-888-283-8806.

Alcohol and other drug treatment

Most people who use alcohol or other drugs do not end up with a problem or dependency. But some do, and many people who come for treatment for alcohol or other drug use problems (also called substance use problems) also have mental health problems.

Treatment for substance use problems is usually based on an abstinence or harm-reduction model. Abstinence programs require you to stop all use of the problem drug. Harm reduction programs offer a greater range of possibilities. You might not cut out drug use altogether, but cut back on the amount you use and decide to use the drug more appropriately—for example, by not drinking and driving. Harm reduction is viewed as a starting point for people who are not ready to change their behaviour completely.

You can live at home and receive treatment through daytime or evening counselling or by taking part in a day program (which means you go to the treatment centre usually three or more days a week for several weeks). Or you can live at the treatment centre and attend a residential treatment program. Residential treatment can be short-term (up to one month) or long-term (about six weeks to six months).

10

Mutual aid or self-help and other support groups provide added support. These include Alcoholics Anonymous (AA) and Gamblers Anonymous (GA). Family and friends who are affected by the addiction may want to look into mutual support groups such as Al-Anon (for family members of people with alcohol use problems) and Co-Anon (for family members of people with cocaine use problems). In some cases, support groups are available for people of a certain age (e.g., youth or older adults) or people from certain cultural or language groups. However, these specialized groups are more likely to be found in cities or larger communities.

More and more mental health and addiction programs are also providing treatment for people who have both an addiction and mental health problem (referred to as a concurrent disorder). Some community mental health centres, addiction treatment agencies and hospitals offer services for these concurrent disorders.

To find out about alcohol and other drug treatment services that can assess your problem, call the Drug and Alcohol Registry of Treatment (DART) toll-free at 1-800-565-8603 or view their Web site at www.dart.on.ca.

You can also look in the Yellow Pages of your phone book under "Addictions" to find a treatment centre. Or contact an employee (or family) assistance program if your workplace offers one.

10

To learn about drugs and their effects, call the 24-hour Drug, Alcohol and Mental Health Information Line of the Centre for Addiction and Mental Health (CAMH) at 416-595-6111 in Toronto or toll-free at 1-800-463-6273. Taped messages in many different languages discuss various substances, and information sheets can be mailed out to you.

CAMH offers alcohol and other drug treatment services to a variety of diverse populations, including women; youth; lesbian, gay, bisexual, transgendered and transsexuals; aboriginals; and African Canadian and Caribbean Youth. For more information, call (416) 535-8501.

Community information centres

There are about 30 community information centres across Ontario. Community information centres provide information about a wide range of services in your area (e.g., community services, day care, health, immigration, low-income housing, sexual assault and mental health agencies, new immigrant and government services).

> To find a community information centre near you, call 211 in Toronto or (416) 397-4636 if you live outside Toronto. You can also view the 211 Web site at www.211toronto.ca.

10

Getting well and staying well

11

People first diagnosed with a mental health problem may feel that life will never be the same. They may find that their condition disrupts their work, school and home life. And they may feel unable to take on responsibilities or take part in activities. These feelings are natural and understandable. But with effective treatment and support, people often return to their previous lifestyle, responsibilities and activities.

Setting goals and priorities is key to making changes successfully. Your goals and priorities are individual—it is different for every person. Set goals that will challenge you and that will allow you to enjoy and find meaning in what you do. And take some risks—without getting too overwhelmed. Decide how much stress is too much for you and know when to slow down. Finding the right balance can be hard, but it can be learned. Getting better is a process that happens in stages.

It helps to discuss your goals with your family, psychiatrist or other health care professional, such as a social worker or a case manager. Both social workers and case managers can link you with other agencies and services, communicate with your family and other caregivers and keep track of your progress. Part of their job is helping you have the best quality of life possible in the community. That could mean finding housing, school, work, social activities or medical care—or dealing with money issues or other hardships.

Family and friends

An important part of recovery is spending time with loved ones—family, friends, a pet or perhaps your co-workers. These supports can be a great source of comfort. Other times you may want to open up to someone who has no connection to your personal life, such as a therapist.

You must be the judge. People who don't listen and people who criticize or put you down are not supportive. Do you have supportive people in your life? Are your relationships only based on getting support from people or do you like spending time together? Does your friend or family member want to be a support?

Social and recreational activities

Exercising. Seeing movies. Having lunch with friends. Taking a bubble bath. Cooking. Looking at clouds. Drinking herbal tea. Taking up a hobby. Volunteering. There are lots of great, low-cost activities you can do alone or with a companion to feel better!

Here are a few more ideas:

- Find out about social and recreation drop-in centres through your local mental health agency, such as the Canadian Mental Health Association.
- Look for programs offered through community centres and your local parks and recreation department.
- Find out about social groups or associations within your ethnocultural community by picking up a copy of the community newspaper.
- Search the Internet for free things to do in your community or city, or check the events listings in your local community newspaper.
- Visit local attractions such as a scenic route, historic site or museum.
- Get involved in local amateur sports organizations.
- Take part in spiritual activities—this could mean attending a church, synagogue, mosque, temple or other religious institution. Or you

11

may want to try meditation, yoga, tai chi, karate, journal writing, drumming, painting, praying or nature walks.

- Explore your creative side. You can take classes through local community colleges, art schools, boards of education, community centres and sometimes hospital outpatient programs.

In the hospital, there may be a recreation therapist who can assess your recreational or social needs and help you create a plan to satisfy these needs. For example, if you're feeling alone or isolated, the recreational therapist may arrange social outings for you.

Work

We all need and deserve the self-respect that comes from doing something meaningful, whether it is a hobby, recreational activity or volunteer or paid work. It gives us a sense of purpose, connects us to other people, and, if we're lucky, provides the money we need to support ourselves.

Our society places a great value on work. Often the first question people ask when they meet someone is, "What do you do?" It's the way people judge others and, often, the way we identify ourselves.

Not having work can be discouraging and financially stressful. People who are out of work may begin to doubt their abilities and lose their self-confidence.

Some people who have a period of mental health problems recover fully and return to their jobs. Others never have to leave their jobs and continue to work as usual. Still others find that their problem is more constant and serious and that related difficulties—such as a lack of confidence, difficulty remembering or paying attention, anxiety, restlessness and tiredness—make it too difficult to work. Sometimes these are symptoms of the mental health problem. Other times they are due to the side-effects of medication.

11

People who have more than one problem (e.g., a substance use problem or an intellectual or physical disability in addition to a mental health problem) may find it harder to get a meaningful job and keep it. And they often face added discrimination.

TYPES OF WORK

Work can mean having a full-time job, working part-time, doing casual work (work that is neither pre-arranged nor regularly scheduled), being self-employed or doing volunteer work to gain experience and confidence in an area that interests you.

Volunteer work is often useful if you have been out of the workplace and need recent work experience and references. It is also an opportunity to find out if you need more training. Casual work is a source of additional income—for instance, for people who receive Canada Pension Plan Disability or Ontario Disability Support Program benefits.

Another option is working with an alternative business. Alternative businesses are started up and managed entirely by consumer/survivors. Employees have the opportunity to work flexible or part-time hours and receive skills training and mentorship (guidance and teaching). They are expected to participate in all business matters and are paid a fair market value for their work. The Ontario Council of Alternative Businesses (OCAB) provides support to consumer/survivor groups that want to set up their own business. Alternative businesses employ more than 800 people across Ontario.

11

For more information about creating an alternative business or working in one and for business contacts, call OCAB at (416) 504-1693 in Toronto. Their Web site is www.icomm.ca/ocab.

For more information on how to approach economic development strategies, you can also contact the Ontario Peer Development Initiative. *(See Consumer/survivor initiatives in Section 10, p. 77.)*

REDUCING JOB STRESS

Many aspects of today's workplaces can contribute to anxiety and depression—everything from job insecurity and intense competition to long hours and contract work.

If you have a job, but worry that the effects of job stress may be making a health problem worse, you may want to consider asking for changes in your workplace or work schedule. These are called workplace accommodations. Depending on your needs, accommodations could mean changes in the workplace (e.g., a quieter office) or changes in how you do the work (e.g., taking more frequent breaks or time off to attend doctor's appointments, changes in job duties, working from home, or receiving more individual supervision or direction). Accommodations are made as long as you can still do the important, central tasks of the job.

In a small organization, approach your immediate supervisor directly about an accommodation; in a large organization, contact your occupational health and safety department or employment (and family) assistance program (EAP or EFAP) first. You may have to tell your boss that you have a mental health problem. This decision should be made carefully. Weigh the possibility of getting special accommodations with the possibility that your supervisor may view you differently as a person and as an employee.

EAPs and EFAPs are programs that an employer provides to its employees, usually for free. EAPs offer a range of mental health services, such as individual, family and marriage counselling and help with alcohol and other drug problems, legal and financial troubles, workplace conflict and other stress-related problems.

11

WORK SUPPORTS

Various income benefit programs offer employment (job) support. This support could include job coaching, computer training and paying transportation costs to attend the training.

- **Ontario Disability Support Program (ODSP)** provides ODSP employment supports without requiring that you be receiving ODSP income benefits. You can receive these supports when you are working: for instance, if you are having trouble keeping your job because of a disability. Supports include specialized equipment, training to use the equipment, people to interpret and take notes, job training, transportation during job training, and job coaching.

  For more information, contact your local ODSP office. Or view the Web site www.cfcs.gov.on.ca/CFCS/en/programs/IES/OntarioDisabilitySupport Program/default.htm.

- **Employment Insurance (EI)** work supports are available to anyone in Canada. Work supports include use of faxes, photocopiers, computers (including Internet access) and job banks. Depending on the office and location, you may be able to get employment counselling and workshops on topics such as writing a resumé and learning job search methods.

  For more information, contact Human Resources Development Canada toll-free at 1-800-206-7218. For a list of Human Resource Centre Canada offices, view the Human Resources Development Canada (HRDC) Web site at www.hrdc-drhc.gc.ca.

- **Ontario Works (OW),** formerly welfare, requires that you take part in an OW activity, such as employment support. (However, exceptions are made if you have younger than school-aged children or medical problems.) Employment supports include academic upgrading, English as a Second Language (ESL) classes and other services to help you find work.

  While involved in an OW employment support program, you may also be eligible for child care expenses and transportation to attend the program.

11

For more information about getting support, contact a caseworker through OW. To find your local OW office, call 211 in Toronto or (416) 397-4636 outside Toronto. Or view the Web site at www.cfcs.gov.on.ca/CFCS/en/programs/IES/OntarioWorks/default.htm.

- **Canada Pension Plan (CPP) Disability Vocational Rehabilitation Program** includes various services to help people receiving CPP disability benefits return to work. A vocational rehabilitation specialist works one-on-one with you on a return-to-work rehabilitation plan. You may also benefit from the program's job search skills, support for retraining costs and one-on-one guidance about your work needs and goals.

  For more information, call Human Resources Development Canada toll-free at 1-800-461-3422.

- **Workplace Safety and Insurance Board (WSIB)**, formerly the Worker's Compensation Board (WCB), supports people who have had a work-related injury or illness. This includes:

  - *traumatic mental stress*—a strong, severe reaction to something sudden and unexpected that happens in the workplace or
  - *psychotraumatic disability*—having a mental health problem that results indirectly from an injury or accident at work or a condition that was caused by the work-related injury.

The disability has to have occurred within five years of the injury or within five years of the last surgical procedure. You cannot receive WSIB benefits for traumatic mental stress that results from the employer's work decisions or actions: for instance, if you are laid off, demoted or transferred.

WSIB provides 85 per cent of your net (after deductions) average income before the accident, helps with health care and offers various work supports. They include return-to-work programs involving

11

changes to your job, job market re-entry assessments, job search skills and financial assistance for post-secondary education or other schooling.

> For more information on WSIB, call 1-800-387-0750 or see the listing of phone numbers and addresses of local WSIB offices on the WSIB Web site at www.wsib.on.ca.

Speak with a local mental health agency (e.g., your local CMHA office) about work supports in your area. Or ask your health care provider to refer you to an employee support program.

(For more information about these programs, see Income benefits on p. 103. For information on vocational programs, see Learning and developing skills below.)

Learning and developing skills

Many people develop a mental health problem between ages 15 and 30, a time when they may be finishing secondary school or taking a post-secondary education program.

People with mental health problems succeed in their education like everyone else but mental health difficulties can affect learning. For instance, people with mental health problems may not be treated well by other students. They may fear failure, feel tired and have problems with some thought processes: focusing attention and thoughts, remembering things in the short-term, thinking and arguing critically, and solving problems. Some people may experience a crisis related to their condition, which could interrupt their studies.

ACCOMMODATIONS

In Ontario high schools, students with behavioural and emotional problems can receive special education through the Individual Education Plan.

However, services for children and youth with mental health problems are very limited in the schools.

Some Ontario universities and community colleges have offices where students with mental health problems can get accommodations, or supports, to help them continue their studies; however, these services may also be limited. The name of the office to go to varies; for instance, it could be called the disability office, accessibility services or special needs office.

These offices can help students get accommodations such as:

• writing exams or tests in a separate location from other students
• having a longer time to write exams or assignments or
• dropping a course after the official deadline without charges.

Students can also get help to access other school services, such as the finance department, tutoring or mental health services. While you can approach a disability office at any time in the school year, contacting them early will mean that your request for an accommodation may be processed faster if you experience a crisis.

LEARNING AND SKILLS PROGRAMS

Some programs will help you upgrade your skills and increase your confidence:

• **Skills training programs** are offered through community and private colleges, universities and high school upgrading services. A local community centre or library may also offer skills training (e.g., computer training for people with low-income) or provide computer time free.
• **Supported education programs** help people with mental health problems prepare to return to school or work. These programs are often offered at community colleges. Classes may include assertiveness training, communication, stress management and academic courses.

11

- **Vocational programs** support your goals to return to work. They can help you rebuild your work skills and self-confidence and find jobs that fit your abilities and needs. These programs offer services such as vocational (job) assessment, career counselling, aptitude (capabilities and skills) testing, job search skills and on-the-job training.

Drug benefits

Psychiatric drugs sometimes cost a lot, but various benefit programs exist that will cover some or all of your medication costs. If you feel that you cannot afford medications, discuss this with your doctor, pharmacist or caseworker. They may have helpful suggestions.

The Ontario government does not cover all prescriptions automatically. Some drugs are only covered for a specific use (e.g., bupropion is covered for use as an antidepressant but not when used by someone to stop smoking). You may have to try other less expensive medications first. If they do not work or have too many side-effects, then the cost of the more expensive or alternative drugs may be covered.

You may be eligible for the following:

- **Ontario's Drug Benefit Program** covers many prescription drugs for people 65 years of age and over and people living on disability or welfare benefits. The program includes a:

  - *Deductible Program* for people aged 65 and over with higher incomes. You pay $100 every year up front (deductible), and then $6.11 for every prescription after that. Everyone automatically receives this benefit at age 65. Pharmacists can submit the claims automatically if they have your health card.

  - *Co-Payment Program* for people aged 65 and over with lower incomes and people receiving support from Ontario Works (OW) or the Ontario Disability Support Program (ODSP). (See p. 103.) Each prescription can be filled for up to $2.

To take part, your income or combined income (with your spouse or partner) must be below a certain amount. Applications are available at your local pharmacy. If you are aged 65 and over and are approved for coverage, give your pharmacist your health card number and your claims will be submitted automatically. If you are on OW or ODSP, you will need to show your drug eligibility card.

To find out more about who can use these programs, call the Seniors Information Line of the Ministry of Health and Long-Term Care toll-free at 1-888-405-0405.

- The **Trillium Drug Program** is an Ontario government drug benefit program. It is aimed at people who have no medical insurance, only limited benefits and/or people who take medications that are very costly in view of their income. Anyone with a valid Ontario health card can use the program. The deductible (amount you pay out first) varies depending on your income or combined income (with your spouse or partner) and the number of people in your family. The deductible is roughly four per cent of your household net income.

After you have paid the deductible, prescriptions cost $2 each. However, as with Ontario's Drug Benefit Program, not all drugs are covered. Applications are available at your local pharmacy.

Call the Ministry of Health and Long-Term Care toll-free at 1-800-575-5386 for more information about the Trillium Drug Program.

11

- If you have a **private health plan** (e.g., a health plan organized through your workplace or Blue Cross), check to see which prescription drugs and what percentage of their costs are covered for you and your family members.

Your pharmacist may not charge the $2 administrative fee to fill a prescription. Pick up your prescriptions in person, so you can ask your pharmacist any questions about the medications. If necessary, some pharmacies will deliver to your home without charge. Look around for a pharmacy that meets your needs.

Legal help

The laws around clients' rights may be difficult to understand, even to people who work in the mental health system. Various brochures and booklets are available to help you know your rights.

- **Community Legal Education Ontario (CLEO)** is a community legal clinic that provides legal information in clear language that may interest people with low incomes and other disadvantaged groups. To order materials from CLEO, view their Web site at www.cleo.on.ca or call them at (416) 408-4420.

- Get a copy of ***Rights and Responsibilities: Mental Health and the Law*** to help you understand laws around mental health issues. *Rights and Responsibilities* is very detailed. The laws it describes may be hard to understand, but it is easier to read than the actual laws! The booklet is put out by the Ministry of Health and Long-Term Care.

  > You can read the full text of *Rights and Responsibilities* on the Consent and Capacity Board Web site at www.ccboard.on.ca. The Ministry provides more information on its Web site at www.gov.on.ca/health.

11

You can call on people who will advocate for you (speak for you and stand up for your rights) and provide you with information about your rights:

- The **Psychiatric Patient Advocate Office (PPAO)** provides rights advice, advocacy services and information on the rights of clients and people looking for mental health services. This includes giving information to clients, families, hospital staff and the community about clients' legal and civic rights. Rights advisers and patient advocates are located in all current and former provincial psychiatric hospitals.

The PPAO can be reached at (416) 327-7000 in Toronto or toll-free at 1-800-578-2343. Or view their Web site at www.ppao.gov.on.ca. For more information about the rights of psychiatric clients, get a free copy of the PPAO's booklet *Psychiatric Patients' Rights under Ontario Health Law.*

QUESTION: What can I do if I have a complaint about the care I have received from a particular health care worker?

ANSWER: The answer really depends on where you are living and your complaint. If you are a client at a psychiatric facility or hospital in Ontario, you can contact the Psychiatric Patient Advocate Office (PPAO). Or find out if there is a client relations office or patient representative that handles your complaints at the hospital. If the complaint is with a community agency or clinic, there won't be a patient advocate. However, certain health care workers, such as a case manager or social worker, could advocate for you. You could also report the problem to the health care worker's employer (e.g., a unit director or a supervisor).

If the complaint is against your therapist, you should contact the complaints department of the governing or regulatory college your therapist belongs to. Usually, a complaint needs to be in writing and must be sent to the registrar or complaints department of the college.

11

For more information, contact the PPAO for a copy of their brochure *How to Complain Against Health and Social Service Practitioners.*

QUESTION: Can I see my file?

ANSWER: Clients in a psychiatric facility can ask to look at and copy their clinical record by filling out a Form 28, which they can get from the health records department of the facility. However, the hospital can try to hold back all or part of your record if you are considered at potential risk to yourself or others. To do this, the hospital must apply for permission to the Consent and Capacity Board. You will get notice of this application, and you have the right to participate in the Board hearing, with or without legal representation.

If you want to see your therapy records and you are receiving therapy outside of a psychiatric hospital, you can write a letter to the therapist requesting your records. Or ask the therapist in person if you can see them.

- **ARCH: A Legal Resource Centre for Persons with Disabilities** is a community legal clinic that serves anyone with a disability, whether it is physical, developmental, mental or emotional. ARCH provides a variety of services, including:
  - free, confidential legal advice and referrals
  - legal representation for precedent-setting (model) cases
  - public legal education (a worker will come and speak to your group about a particular legal issue relating to disabilities)
  - *ARCH Alert,* a newsletter about subjects related to disability and the law.

  ARCH can be reached by calling (416) 482-8255 in Toronto or toll-free at 1-866-482-2724. Their TTY line is (416) 482-1254. You can view their Web site at www.arch-online.org.

If you need legal advice, there are a number of ways to find a lawyer who knows mental health law:

- Talk to family members and friends to see if they know someone.

11

- Contact a community agency, such as a counselling service or women's shelter, to see if they know someone who can help you.
- Check the Yellow Pages of your phone book under "Lawyer" or contact the Lawyer Referral Service offered by the Law Society of Upper Canada (Ontario). Note: There is an automatic charge of $6 for contacting this service at 1-900-565-4577. People in jail, people under 18 or people in crisis situations (e.g., domestic abuse) can call (416) 947-3330 in Toronto or toll-free at 1-800-268-8326. The referral service gives you up to a half-hour free consultation, which includes referring you to a lawyer who's best suited to help with your concerns and needs.

> If you need help to pay for a lawyer, contact Legal Aid Ontario to find out if you can use their services and, if so, how to apply. Call them at (416) 979-1446 in Toronto or toll-free at 1-800-668-8258. Or visit their Web site at www.legalaid.on.ca. *(For information on diversion programs, see Forensic services, p. 68, in Section 8.)*

Housing

We all need comfortable, safe, affordable housing, a place we can live with dignity—not just a house but a home.

Many people will comfortably continue to live where they've always lived. But some people will need to make changes. If you need housing, various options exist for people with a mental health problem. You can find an apartment or house where you can live independently or with varying levels of support from workers who will come to your home. Or you can live in a home where you have support with day-to-day living.

If you have been an inpatient in a psychiatric hospital or unit, a social worker or caseworker may talk to you and members of your family about living arrangements. You may be able to return home, go to a group home or find a room or apartment where you can live on your own. It is common for people to try one living plan and then another

11

to find the one that suits them best. For instance, you may find that a more supportive environment is important early on in your recovery, but you might prefer to live independently at a later stage. Ask about all the options that are available in the community.

CHOOSING THE BEST HOUSING

What you choose will depend on your needs as well as what is available when you are looking. Here are some questions to help you choose the most appropriate housing:

- How much can you pay? (Prepare a budget.)
- Do you like the neighbourhood? Is it safe?
- Is the place in good condition?
- How much support do you need?
- Is there shopping close by? Public transportation? Are you close to a mental health agency or worker?
- Do you want to live alone or with others? If you choose to live with other people, will you be compatible with them in the home?

There are housing workers in the community who can assess your housing needs and tell you about the housing and supports that are available. You may face a waiting period before the type of housing you want becomes available.

TYPES OF HOUSING

The range of housing choices varies greatly between communities—with far less available to First Nations and other isolated communities. Here are the five main types of housing:

- **Private market housing** refers to a home that is privately owned. There are no government subsidies and the rent is not based on your income. This includes:
  - rooms, flats, apartments (in a house or apartment building) or houses. It is usually cheaper to live with other people than to live alone. If you want to live alone or choose to share a place

with other(s), you could check the For Rent listings in the Classifieds section of newspapers. If you prefer to find a place where people are looking for a housemate, check the Shared Accommodations listings under Classifieds. (Shared accommodation usually means having your own bedroom and sharing the rest of the space in the house or apartment.) You could also look for signs on public bulletin boards (e.g., in laundromats or grocery stores) or windows of houses in the area where you would like to live.

– rooming or boarding houses. Both rooming and boarding houses involve living together in one house or building, and often sharing rooms with someone else. Rooming houses do not include meals; boarding houses do include meals.

• **Social housing** is housing that is partly paid for by government or charges rent geared to income. In this kind of housing, the rent will never be more than 30 per cent of your income. For this reason, many people on social assistance (e.g., Ontario Works or Ontario Disability Support Plan) choose this option. However, there are often long waiting lists—sometimes as long as eight to 10 years.

> In Toronto, you can call Toronto Social Housing Connections (416) 392-6111 to find out about all rent-geared-to-income places in the city. There is no central number for social housing outside Toronto.

• **Supportive housing** is housing where there are support workers in the home who work for the housing provider. The support varies depending on what you need. There could be no support, on-call support, weekly or daily support or 24-hour-a-day support. To get into supportive housing, you need to meet certain conditions: have a diagnosis of a mental disorder for a minimum length of time or have been admitted to a psychiatric facility a minimum number of times or for a minimum amount of time.

11

Most supportive housing (e.g., a boarding home, a group home or a co-op) involves sharing living space. However, there are some apartments where you can live on your own.

- **Supported housing** differs from supportive housing. With supported housing, the support worker provides care and services from outside the home. People living in supported housing tend to need much less support and can live more independently than people in supportive housing. Supported housing could be a social housing coalition or any other housing environment that provides staff from a community agency. Support workers could be:

  - visiting homemakers who come in for about an hour a day to help with chores like laundry and cleaning (This service is not easy to get.)
  - case managers or support workers who spend most of their time helping the client with living skills, such as learning to use the local transit system or learning to cook, prepare a budget and shop or
  - nurses who give medication and provide support and counselling.

- **Emergency housing** includes shelters and hostels. It is set up as temporary housing for people in crisis. The people who use shelters and hostels generally have no home or their homes have become unsafe (e.g., people who are living on the street, refugees or new immigrants awaiting housing, women who have been abused). Many shelters provide services to specific groups of people: women only, families, women and children, single men only or youth). *(See Safe houses and shelters, p. 74, in Section 9.)*

11

For information about landlord and tenant laws, call the Ontario Rental Housing Tribunal's toll-free number at 1-888-332-3234, or view their Web site at www.orht.gov.on.ca.

Community Legal Education Ontario (CLEO) offers free, easy-to-read information on such topics as rent increases, maintenance and repairs and care homes. To order materials from CLEO, view their Web site at www.cleo.on.ca or call (416) 408-4420.

If you are looking for housing but don't have a telephone where some-one can reach you, some drop-in centres or community facilities will let you use their address or phone number as a temporary contact. Some may even set up a voice mail message system for you.

Income benefits

Many people with mental health problems maintain their job and in-come levels. For others, it is a struggle and they may find themselves in need of income support. The income programs listed below have different applications, conditions and requirements. They may also have long waiting times.

TYPES OF BENEFITS

These are all income benefits not related to work that you may qualify for if you have a mental health problem. *(For work-related benefits, see Work supports on p. 89.)*

- **Ontario Works (OW)**, formerly GWA or general welfare assistance, provides financial help and employment support for people who are able to work but unable to find a job, or unable due to medical problems. OW helps people who are applying for Ontario Disability Support Program benefits but need money right away. You can apply directly at the municipal office closest to where you live or by calling toll-free at 1-888-465-4478. You may be able to apply by phone and bring the required support documents to the office. A caseworker at your local office can provide more information.

- **Ontario Disability Support Program (ODSP)**, formerly known as Family Benefits or FBA, is funded by the Ministry of Community, Family and Children's Services. ODSP provides financial assistance to people who have a substantial mental or physical impairment or disability that is expected to last a year or more and affects the person's ability to handle work or daily living. Financial assistance is available up to $930 per month for a single person and up to

11

$1,417 for a family of two or more. You may also be able to get other help, such as public transit tickets. Ask about all possible types of financial help.

You can apply for ODSP directly at the Ministry of Community, Family and Children's Services office or your local OW (social services) office if you need money immediately. The application includes forms that must be filled out by your doctor or another health care professional.

– *STEP* is an ODSP benefit that allows you to have more money if you choose to work. Through STEP, you can keep your full ODSP cheque and earn up to $160 per month at a job, if you are single, and up to $235 per month at a job, if you have a family. If you make more than these amounts, your ODSP cheque is reduced. Even if your income is high enough that you are taken off ODSP, you may still qualify to receive health benefits if you have high medication costs. If you lose your job for any reason, you can get back on ODSP.

– *Community Start-Up Benefit (CSUB)* is an ODSP/OW benefit of up to $799 to help you with costs to set up a new home (e.g., buying furniture, moving costs, rent deposit). To get CSUB, you must qualify for ODSP or OW. And you must be moving either because your current home is unsafe (e.g., you have an abusive partner) or you are leaving an institution, such as a psychiatric hospital, group home or prison. To get the CSUB, you will have to give your OW (social services) or ODSP caseworker an item-by-item list of costs to move and set up your housing.

– *Personal Needs Allowance (PNA)* of $112 per month ($3.75 per day) is available to people who receive ODSP (and their dependants) if they are in a provincial psychiatric hospital or one of various other facilities. This money is meant for personal spending and costs for items such as clothing, school tuition, hygiene products and nutritional supplements that are not provided by the facility.

- **Canada Pension Plan (CPP) Disability Benefits** is a program funded by the Canadian government and run by the Income Security Programs of Human Resources Development Canada. This plan provides income benefits to people (and their dependent children) who:

  – have contributed to CPP for a minimum qualifying period
  – have a severe, continuing physical or mental disability, as defined by CPP legislation and
  – are between the ages of 18 and 65.

  You must apply in writing. To get an application kit, call toll-free at 1-800-277-9914. If you have a hearing or speech impairment and use a TDD/TTY device, call 1-800-255-4786. You can also view the Human Resources Development Canada Web site at www.hrdc-drhc.gc.ca/isp.

TIPS ON APPLYING

- Before going to the office, make sure that you have all the right identification, which may include birth certificate; passport; proof of citizenship, for immigrants who have become Canadian citizens; record of landing, for permanent residents or immigrants; social insurance number; health card. And have all the papers ready that you need (e.g., current bank statements, proof of housing or shelter and expenses, proof of income from any source).
- Find out when the office is open and—if possible—the least busy time to go.
- If you are calling a phone line, try first thing in the morning and avoid lunch hour.
- If you have an appointment about your application, be on time by planning to be early, in case of problems with transportation.
- Contact a community legal clinic for help if you have been denied ODSP and need help to appeal the decision.

11

Help for families

12

There are two reasons why you, as a family member, may access mental health services: to find treatment and support for someone in your family who has a mental health problem or to get information and support for yourself.

The effect on family members

When someone has a serious mental health problem, it is natural for the person's family members to feel worried and stressed. You may be mourning a change triggered by a newly diagnosed mental health problem in someone close to you. Or you may be exhausted with trying to help your family member, at the sacrifice of your own needs being met. It is common for family members to feel confused or fearful about what the future holds—or angry or guilty about times they have spent with the family member. Some people lose touch with their own network of friends, which can make them feel isolated and alone.

Often people take a long time to realize how emotionally and physically worn out they have become. The stress can lead to sleeping poorly and feeling exhausted or irritable all the time.

If you are experiencing this stress yourself, don't despair. Seeing the signs is the first step to looking after your own physical and mental health. Finding your own limits and making time for yourself are keys to self-care. Caring for your own needs includes creating a support system of friends and family you can rely on. Think about people you might want to share your thoughts and feelings with. Mental health problems are hard for some people to understand. Open up to people who will support you. And help others by sharing the information and knowledge you have gained. Also, make sure that—along with your own needs—you focus on the needs of other family members who may be in the same situation.

There may be times when people's mental health problems cause them to behave dangerously, but violence is not common among people with mental health problems. In fact, they are far more likely to be the victims of violent or aggressive behaviour than to commit violence. However, when someone who has a mental health problem is aggressive, their actions will often be directed toward the people close to them.

Care for families

There are many practical ways to take care of your own needs:

- Learn as much as you can about your family member's mental health problem. You can get *information* on mental health issues and policies through family support programs, hospitals and organizations that focus on specific disorders, such as the Schizophrenia Society of Ontario and the Mood Disorders Association of Ontario. (*For contact information, see Appendix B.*) You can also find out about individual family support projects or programs by contacting your local Canadian Mental Health Association office.

- Join a *support group or support program* for family members: you can discuss your feelings, get support and learn from others in a similar situation. Family support groups or programs often focus on a specific problem (e.g., schizophrenia or bipolar disorder). In addition to groups for all family members, there are special groups just for spouses, children or parents of people with mental health problems. Some family support programs also have staff or trained volunteers who can give individual support. You can find support groups and

12

programs through hospitals, community mental health agencies and self-help organizations. Contact specific family support groups through the Schizophrenia Society of Ontario and the Mood Disorders Association of Ontario. Find out how you can get involved. (*See Self-help groups, p. 80, in Section 10.*)

- Find out about the many other services available to you: from marriage or family therapy to massage, naturopathy or opportunities for creative expression. (*See Section 4: About therapy, p. 27, and Section 6: Natural healing, p. 51.*)

- Look into *educational groups* that help family members and friends understand what the person with a mental health problem is going through. You can learn about symptoms and treatment (e.g., medication or natural therapies). And you can learn about how to help someone you care about and limits to the help you can give. Educational groups may be offered at the hospital or community agency where your family member is being treated. Some self-help organizations have regular education meetings. Think about finding your own therapist. (*See Section 4: About therapy, p. 27.*)

CHALLENGE: You do not have anyone to care for your children while you go to an appointment. (This can be a particular worry for single parents.)

SUGGESTION: Find out if child care is offered through the program or if you can bring your children with you.

How you can help

SUPPORT YOUR FAMILY MEMBER TO GET HELP

Someone who is moderately depressed or anxious is more likely to agree to get help without needing to be talked into it. But a person with a severe, ongoing mental health problem may refuse treatment. The person may not believe there is a problem. He or she may want to avoid the mental health system because of a bad experience or may feel that treatment will not make a difference.

You may try over and over again to convince your family member to take his or her medication or talk to a doctor. But trying to coax and persuade sometimes leads to arguments and continuing conflict. Although you may be very close to your family member, your views may not be welcome. The person may shut you out. Sometimes it helps to have someone else you trust talk to your family member.

TAKE ACTION

There are other ways you can help yourself and your family member.

- Familiarize yourself with parts of the *Mental Health Act*; for instance, the forms that have to be filled out for a mandatory psychiatric assessment and possible hospitalization. Family support programs are also a good place to find this kind of information. *(See Appendix C, Forms 1 and 2 and information below about calling the police.)*

- Suggest to your family member that he or she consider making a power of attorney for personal care or property in the event that he or she may become incapable of making decisions about personal care (including treatment) or money and other property. *(For information on contacting a lawyer, see Legal help, p. 96, in Section 11. For more information on mental health laws, see Section 13: Understanding your rights, p. 113.)*

- Write a journal with details of your family member's problem. This could include the history of the problem (e.g., when the problem started, how it began and progressed, how many times he or she had symptoms and what they were) as well as a record of treatment (e.g. hospitalizations, medications and a list of the health care professionals who treated your family member). It may help to prepare the history with another family member; different people may have had different experiences or may remember things differently.

Confidentiality laws prevent professionals from sharing family information about an adult client without that person's consent, but family members are allowed to provide information. So a journal can be very helpful.

12

- Prepare a crisis plan if your family member or someone close to you has been in a crisis, in case of another emergency. Keep this plan near the phone or somewhere else where it is easy to find.

  A crisis plan contains all the information that would be important to have should there be a crisis. For instance, write down the names and phone numbers of:

  - the hospital nearest you
  - a mobile crisis unit (see *Mobile crisis units and services, p. 73, in Section 9*) and
  - a community relations or other contact person at the local police department.

Making contact and informing the local police about your family member's situation will help if a crisis occurs, especially when there is a continuing problem.

- If your family member is in conflict with the law, find out more about court diversion programs and other mental health services in the court system. (*See Section 8: More intensive and specialized support, p. 65.*)
- If you think your family member might harm him- or herself or others, you might want to consider having your family member put in a hospital. You can contact a doctor, a justice of the peace or the police.

  - A doctor can make a house call to assess if your family member can be taken to a psychiatric facility for a period of up to 72 hours (three days) for a more complete assessment under Form 1 of the Ontario *Mental Health Act.*
  - A justice of the peace can issue a Form 2 for a psychiatric assessment authorizing the police to take your family member to the hospital. This is based on a sworn statement from you. Your family member does not have to have seen a doctor. However, the Form 2 only requires that your family member be brought to the psychiatric

12

facility for an assessment. The person only stays in the hospital if a doctor issues a Form 1.

To contact a justice of the peace in Toronto, call (416) 327-5179. To find a justice of the peace outside of Toronto, contact your local courthouse.

– The police are authorized to take someone to the hospital for an assessment if the police or someone else, such as a family member, have seen the person behaving dangerously as a result of a mental health problem or if they have a completed Form 1 or Form 2. *(See Appendix C for more details about Form 1 and Form 2.)*

- Prepare a list of questions before you meet with the people who are helping your family member. The following will give you an idea of the questions you might ask, depending on whether your family member is already in a hospital or is still being assessed:
    – Are there any resources to help me cope?
    – Who will assess (or who has assessed) my family member?
    – When will we know how long my family member will be kept in hospital?
    – What are visiting hours? Can children come?
    – Can I bring food or gifts?
    – Can I meet the social worker and primary care nurse to discuss plans for leaving the hospital?
    – Can I be involved in my family member's care team?
    – Will you contact me before my family member is discharged?

(For information about how someone can admit themselves to a hospital, or about admitting someone to hospital against their will, see Section 13: Understanding your rights, p. 113.)

12

Understanding your rights

13

Ontario mental health laws

There are three main acts that outline your rights with respect to mental health services. The *Mental Health Act* is a set of rules decided by the Ontario legislature that gives doctors and psychiatric facilities certain powers and gives patients particular rights. These laws apply in general hospital psychiatric units and psychiatric hospitals but not mental health clinics. The *Health Care Consent Act* deals with rules for consenting, or agreeing, to treatment. The *Substitute Decisions Act* deals with how decisions can be made for a person and the appointment of powers of attorney for personal care and property. *(See the Glossary for an explanation of the term power of attorney.)*

The *Mental Health Act* deals with many inpatient issues, including:

- when someone can be taken and admitted to a psychiatric facility involuntarily
- how a person can be kept in the hospital
- who can see a patient's records in the facility, and how to arrange to see them
- a patient's right to information and right to appeal being involuntarily admitted, held in a facility, denied access to records and so on.

Being admitted to hospital

VOLUNTARY ADMISSION

Most people are admitted voluntarily to a psychiatric facility. They choose to enter the hospital for help with a problem. To be admitted voluntarily for care, you can get a doctor's recommendation or go to the emergency department of a psychiatric or general hospital or a local distress centre. You will be admitted if you need observation, care and treatment provided by an inpatient psychiatric facility.

INVOLUNTARY ADMISSION

Admitting someone against his or her wishes is a much more difficult situation for everyone concerned. The law identifies various ways to admit a person to a hospital as an involuntary, or certified, patient. The person must be seen to be a danger to him- or herself or to others, or at risk of serious physical impairment due to a mental health problem. A person can also be admitted involuntarily *if* the following are all true:

- The person received treatment for a mental health problem before.
- The person showed clinical improvement as the result of the treatment.
- Based on the person's history and condition, it is likely that the person will cause harm to him- or herself or others, or to suffer substantial mental or physical deterioration or serious physical impairment.
- The person has been found to be incapable of consent and a substitute decision-maker (SDM) *(see definition on p. 136)* consents to treatment on his or her behalf AND
- The person is not suitable for informal or voluntary admission.

You can become an involuntary patient (required to stay in the hospital) if you meet the criteria or conditions described above. How long you have to stay in the hospital depends on how long you continue to meet the involuntary criteria or conditions. The *Mental Health Act* requires that certain forms must be used to admit patients and keep them in the hospital involuntarily, and to let them know about their rights. *(To look at some commonly used forms, see Appendix C.)*

13

If you are an involuntary client, you cannot leave the hospital unless permitted under conditions set by a doctor. If you disagree with being committed to (or kept in) the hospital, you can apply to the Consent and Capacity Board to have the doctor's decision reviewed. Members of this board are not part of the health care team responsible for your care. If you want legal representation (a lawyer) at the hearing, Legal Aid Ontario may be able to cover the costs.

(For more information about rights advice, see Legal help, p. 96, in Section 11.)

Consenting to or refusing treatment

The *Health Care Consent Act* sets out the rules for making decisions about treatment.

WHEN YOU ARE CAPABLE OF MAKING DECISIONS ABOUT YOUR TREATMENT

You have the right to make a decision about your treatment if you are capable of doing so. You are considered capable of making a decision about treatment if you are able:

- to understand the information that is relevant to the decision about the treatment and
- to appreciate the likely consequences of consenting to or refusing the treatment (or of not making the decision at all).

While in the hospital, you can refuse psychiatric treatment if you are considered mentally capable to decide on treatment. All people have the right to get information from their doctor before consenting to treatment. That information should include:

- the nature of the treatment
- expected benefits of the treatment
- important risks of the treatment
- important side-effects of the treatment

13

- other approaches that could be taken and
- what will probably happen if you don't have the treatment.

WHEN YOU ARE NOT CAPABLE OF MAKING DECISIONS
ABOUT YOUR TREATMENT

If you are found incapable of making treatment decisions, a substitute decision-maker (SDM) is asked to make decisions for you. The SDM has to make choices based on what you said you would want when you were capable. If you didn't express any wishes, the SDM must act in your "best interests."

An SDM may be a person's guardian, a power of attorney for personal care, someone appointed by the Consent and Capacity Board or a family member. If no one is available to act as an SDM, the Office of the Public Guardian and Trustee assumes this role. *(See Public guardian and trustee in the Glossary.)*

> For more information or to get power of attorney forms, view the Web site of the Ministry of the Attorney General at www.attorneygeneral.jus.gov.on.ca and click on Power of Attorney. Or call the Office of the Public Guardian and Trustee at (416) 314-2803 in Toronto or toll-free at 1-800-366-0335.

WHEN YOU ARE NOT ABLE TO MANAGE YOUR FINANCES

If you become a patient in a psychiatric facility or unit, your doctor may find that you are incapable of managing your money and your property. To be judged "incapable of managing your property" means you are not able to understand important information about your finances and you cannot appreciate the consequences of making or not making financial decisions.

13

Unless you already have a guardian of property or you have made a power of attorney for property that states who will make money and property decisions for you, the Public Guardian and Trustee (PGT) becomes your guardian of property under the *Mental Health Act* and makes those decisions. The PGT is a government worker who will manage your property by making sure that money owed to you is paid and your bills and other expenses are paid. The PGT may let another person (e.g., a family member) take over responsibility if the person shows that he or she has a plan for managing your property in a way that is fair and appropriate.

If you think there is a risk that you might be found incapable of managing your finances, you can set up a power of attorney for property to allow someone you trust to take care of these responsibilities (such as paying your mortgage or credit cards). For instance, someone with bipolar disorder or schizophrenia may appoint someone they trust to have power of attorney if necessary.

If you are found to be incapable of managing your property or finances, and you have not already made a continuing power of attorney while you were capable, the court may select a guardian of property for you.

> For more information and to get the necessary forms, view the Web site of the Ministry of the Attorney General at www.attorneygeneral.jus.gov.on.ca and click on Power of Attorney. Or call the Office of the Public Guardian and Trustee at (416) 314-2803 in Toronto or toll-free at 1-800-366-0335.

Community treatment orders

In December 2000, laws about community treatment orders (CTOs) were added to the *Mental Health Act*. A CTO is a legal order, issued by a doctor, and consented to by the person or his or her substitute decision-maker. The CTO outlines the conditions a person with a serious mental health problem must meet to live in the community.

You can be put on a CTO if you have a serious mental illness and meet the following criteria:

13

• You have been an inpatient in a psychiatric unit two or more times or for at least 30 days in the last three years.

- You and others helping with your care (e.g., SDM, doctor) have made a community treatment plan.
- Your doctor has talked with the people named in your treatment plan, and they agree to their part in the plan.
- Your doctor knows that you and your SDM (if you have one) have had the chance to talk with a rights adviser.
- You or your SDM (if you have one) agrees to the plan.
- Your doctor has examined you 72 hours before entering into the plan. He or she also believes that:

  – You will likely become unwell if you do not get treatment or care, and continued supervision in the community. Without this care, your mental illness may cause you to seriously harm your own body or someone else's. Or you could get much worse mentally or physically, or become physically hurt.
  – If you are not now a patient in a psychiatric facility, your doctor believes you meet the criteria for a Form 1.
  – The care, treatment and supervision described in your treatment plan is available in the community.

CTOs are often used for people who come into contact with the mental health system repeatedly. Generally, treatment has worked for them but—for various reasons—they do not continue treatment after leaving the hospital.

CTOs cannot be used to treat people against their will while they are in the community. But if someone does not follow the requirements of the CTO, that person can be brought against their will to see the psychiatrist issuing the CTO and could possibly be hospitalized.

13

If you can't afford to pay for legal services, you can apply for legal aid. For a list of legal aid offices/clinics in your area, view the Legal Aid Ontario Web site at www.legalaid.on.ca.

Appendix A:
1-800 hotlines

In a crisis, call 911. Other emergency numbers are listed at the front of the phone book.

Assaulted Women's Helpline, (416) 863-0511 in Toronto or toll-free at 1-866-863-0511 or TTY 1-866-863-7868, is an anonymous and confidential crisis line for abused and assaulted women in Ontario. They provide crisis counselling, emotional support, safety plans and referrals (eg. for shelters, rape crisis centres, housing, legal services), and interpretation services.

Kids Help Phone, 1-800-668-6868, is a bilingual national telephone counselling service for children and youth. Lines are open 24 hours a day.

Lesbian, Gay, Bi Youth Hotline, 1-800-268-9688, is a provincial hotline for gay, lesbian, bisexual, transexual, transgendered, two-spirited and unsure youth.

Parent Help Line, 1-888-603-9100, is a 24-hour telephone counselling and referral line providing parents with information and support related to parenting issues.

Victim Support Line, 1-888-579-2888, is an Ontario referral service that connects victims of crimes to community services. It is provided by the Attorney General's office.

Appendix B: Resources

Across Boundaries
Contact: (416) 787-3007 in Toronto
Web: www.web.net/~accbound
Across Boundaries provides supports and services to people of colour from various ethnoracial communities who have mental health problems.

American Academy of Child & Adolescent Psychiatry
Web: www.aacap.org

Anxiety Disorders Association of Ontario
Contact: (613) 729-6761 in Ottawa or toll-free at 1-877-308-3843
Web: www.anxietyontario.com

Applied Psychotherapy and Biofeedback
Web: www.aapb.org

ARCH: A Legal Resource Centre for Persons with Disabilities
Contact: (416) 482-8255 in Toronto or toll-free at 1-866-482-2724
  Their TTY line is (416) 482-1254.
Web: www.arch-online.org

Canadian Health Network
Web: www.canadian-health-network.ca

Canadian Mental Health Association, National Office
Contact: (416) 484-7750 in Toronto
Web: www.cmha.ca

Canadian Mental Health Association, Ontario Division
Contact: (416) 977-5580 in Toronto or toll-free at 1-800-875-6213
Web: www.ontario.cmha.ca

Centre for Addiction and Mental Health
Contact: (416) 535-8501 in Toronto
Drug, Alcohol and Mental Health Information Line:
   (416) 595-6111 in Toronto or toll-free at 1-800-463-6273
Web: www.camh.net

Children's Mental Health Ontario
Contact: (416) 921-2109 in Toronto
Web: www.cmho.org

College of Dietitians of Ontario
Contact: (416) 598-1725 in Toronto or toll-free at 1-800-668-4990
Web: www.cdo.on.ca

College of Physicians and Surgeons of Ontario
Contact: (416) 967-2626 (Find a Doctor Service), (416) 967-2603
   (General Inquiries) in Toronto or toll-free at 1-800-268-7096
Web: www.cpso.on.ca

Community Legal Education Ontario (CLEO)
Web: www.cleo.on.ca

Consent and Capacity Board
Web: www.ccboard.on.ca

Consumer Health Information Service
Contact: (416) 393-7056 in Toronto or toll-free at 1-800-667-1999

Dawn Ontario: DisAbled Women's Network Ontario
Contact: (705) 494-9078 in North Bay
Web: http://dawn.thot.net

Dietitians of Canada
Contact: (416) 596-0857 in Toronto
Web: www.dietitians.ca

Distress Centres Ontario
Web: www.dcontario.org

Drug and Alcohol Registry of Treatment (DART)
Contact: (519) 439-0174 in London or toll-free at 1-800-565-8603
Web: www.dart.on.ca

GP Psychotherapy Association (GPPA)
Contact: (416) 410-6644

Human Resources Development Canada
Web: www.hrdc-drhc.gc.ca

Internet Mental Health
Web: www.mentalhealth.com

Lawyer Referral Service of the Law Society of Upper Canada (Ontario)
Contact: 1-900-565-4577—automatic charge of $6

Legal Aid Ontario
Contact: (416) 979-1446 in Toronto or toll-free at 1-800-668-8258
Web: www.legalaid.on.ca

LEGIT—The Lesbian & Gay Immigration Task Force—Canada
Contact: (613) 230-6522 in Ottawa or (416) 944-8801 in Toronto
Web: www.qrd.org/qrd/www/world/immigration/legit.html
LEGIT provides immigration information and support to same-sex partners.

Ministry of the Attorney General
Web: www.attorneygeneral.jus.gov.on.ca

Ministry of Health and Long-Term Care
Contact: (416) 314-5518 in Toronto or toll-free at 1-800-268-1154
Web: ww.gov.on.ca/health/english/program/
mental_health/mentalhealth_mn.html

Mood Disorders Association of Ontario
Contact: (416) 486-8046 in Toronto or toll-free at 1-888-486-8236
Web: www.mooddisorders.on.ca

Motherisk
Contact: (416) 813-6780 in Toronto or the toll-free
Alcohol and Substance Use Helpline at 1-877-327-4636
Web: www.motherisk.org
Motherisk provides information about the effects of alcohol, as well as prescription, over-the-counter and illegal drug use during pregnancy and while breastfeeding.

National Eating Disorder Information Centre
Contact: (416) 340-4156 in Toronto or toll-free at 1-866-633-4220
Web: www.nedic.ca

National Institute of Mental Health
Web: www.nimh.nih.gov

National Network for Mental Health
Contact: (905) 682-2423 in St. Catharines or toll-free at 1-888-406-4663

Office of the Public Guardian and Trustee
Contact: (416) 314-2803 in Toronto or toll-free at 1-800-366-0335

Ontario Association for Marriage and Family Therapy
Contact: (416) 364-2627 in Toronto or toll-free at 1-800-267-2638
Web: www.oamft.on.ca

Ontario Association of Acupuncture and Traditional Chinese Medicine
Contact: (416) 944-2265 in Toronto

Ontario Association of Naturopathic Doctors
Contact: (416) 233-2001 in Toronto or toll-free at 1-877-628-7284
Web: www.oand.org

Ontario Association of Social Workers
Contact: (416) 923-4848 in Toronto
Web: www.oasw.org

Ontario College of Social Workers and Social Service Workers
Web: www.ocswssw.org

Ontario Council of Alternative Businesses (OCAB)
Contact: (416) 504-1693 in Toronto
Web: www.icomm.ca/ocab

Ontario Disability Support Program through the Ministry of Community, Family and Children's Services
Web: www.cfcs.gov.on.ca/CFCS/en/programs/IES/
   OntarioDisabilitySupportProgram/default.htm

Ontario Massage Therapist Association
Contact: (416) 979-2010 in Toronto or toll-free at 1-800-668-2022

Ontario Obsessive Compulsive Disorder Network
Contact: (416) 410-4772 in Toronto
Web: www.oocdn.org

Ontario Peer Development Initiative
Contact: (416) 484-8785 in Toronto or toll-free at 1-866-681-6661
Web: www.opdi.org

Ontario Psychological Association
Contact: (416) 961-0069 in Toronto or toll-free at 1-800-268-0069
Web: www.psych.on.ca

Ontario Rental Housing Tribunal

Contact: toll-free at 1-888-332-3234

Web: www.orht.gov.on.ca

Ontario Self-Help Network (OSHNET) of the Self-Help Resource Centre

Contact: (416) 487-4355 in Toronto or toll-free at 1-888-283-8806

Web: www.selfhelp.on.ca/oshnet.html

Ontario Women's Health Network

Contact: (416) 408-4840 in Toronto

Web: www.owhn.on.ca

Ontario Works

Web: www.cfcs.gov.on.ca/CFCS/en/programs/IES/OntarioWorks/default.htm

Progress Place

Web: www.progressplace.org

This is the first and largest clubhouse in Canada.

PSYCHDIRECT

Web: www.psychdirect.com

This is McMaster University's educational Web site on mental health issues.

Psychiatric Patient Advocate Office (PPAO)

Contact: (416) 327-7000 in Toronto or toll-free at 1-800-578-2343

Web: www.ppao.gov.on.ca

Schizophrenia Society of Canada

Contact: (905) 415-2007 in Toronto or toll-free
  at 1-888-SSC-HOPE (772-4673)

Web: www.schizophrenia.ca

Schizophrenia Society of Ontario

Contact: (416) 449-6830 in Toronto or toll-free at 1-800-449-6367

Web: www.schizophrenia.on.ca

Shelternet

Web: www.shelternet.ca

Shelternet provides a list of shelters for women who have been abused.

Shiatsu Therapy Association of Ontario

Contact: (416) 923-7826 in Toronto or toll-free at 1-877-923-7826

StressFree Net

Web: www.stressfree.com

Telehealth Ontario

Contact: 1-866-797-0000 and TTY is 1-800-387-5559

Web: www.gov.on.ca/health/english/program/
　　　telehealth/telehealth_mn.html

Toronto Social Housing Connections

Contact: (416) 392-6111 in Toronto

211 Toronto

Contact: 211 in Toronto or (416) 397-4636 from outside Toronto

Web: www.211toronto.ca

211 Toronto provides information about community services in Toronto and some surrounding areas.

Please note: Aside from the Centre for Addiction and Mental Health (CAMH) Web site, CAMH does not endorse any of the sites listed above.

Appendix C: Common legal forms

Form 1 (Application for Psychiatric Assessment) can be used to bring someone to a psychiatry facility for an assessment that lasts up to 72 hours (three days). To put someone on a Form 1, a doctor must have personally examined the person within the previous seven days and have reason to believe that the person meets certain tests under the *Mental Health Act. (See Being admitted to hospital, p. 114, in Section 13 for more details about these tests.)*

Form 1 also ensures that another doctor will examine the person with the mental health problem. During the assessment, other mental health professionals (e.g., nurses, psychologists and social workers) may meet with the person and his or her involved family members, friends or caregivers to get additional information.

Form 2 (Order for Examination) is used under the same conditions as the Form 1 but is issued by a justice of the peace. Typically, the Form 2 is used by a person's family or friends when it is not possible for the person to be examined by a doctor. This form allows the police to bring the person to a hospital for a psychiatric assessment. But the form does not authorize the person to be kept at the hospital. If an assessment in hospital is necessary, the examining doctor must then complete a Form 1.

Form 3 (Certificate of Involuntary Admission) is used to admit the person to the hospital against his or her will. A Form 3 cannot be issued by the same doctor who issued the Form 1. The Form 3 means that the person will have to stay in hospital for up to two weeks. The person has a right to have the Consent and Capacity Board quickly review the form.

Form 4 (Certificate of Renewal) is used when a doctor determines that the person must remain in the hospital involuntarily for another month. This certificate can later be renewed so that the person has to stay for another two months (second renewal) or up to three months (third renewal or more). The certificate can be renewed indefinitely. But each time it is renewed, the person can apply for a review by the Consent and Capacity Board.

Form 5 (Change to Voluntary Status) is used when a doctor determines that the person does not need to be kept involuntarily anymore. This form can be completed at any time to end a Form 3 or a Form 4 before it expires. A patient is automatically considered voluntary once his or her certificate expires and another one is not completed.

Form 14 (Consent to the Disclosure, Transmittal or Examination of a Clinical Record) is used when a patient wants to give another person the permission to see or get a copy of his or her clinical record.

Form 28 (Request to Examine or to Copy Clinical Record) is used by a person who wants to get a copy of his or her own clinical record.

These and other forms can be found on the Ministry of Health and Long-Term Care Web site at www.gov.on.ca/health.

Appendix D:
Local contacts

ORGANIZATION	CONTACT

Glossary

Advocates are people who speak for or support someone else and stand up for that person's rights.

Assertive community treatment (ACT) team is a multidisciplinary team (a group of professionals with different areas of expertise) offering intensive case management for people with severe, continuing mental health problems. ACT teams help people who have been hospitalized often and who may need help managing their medication, finding housing, and using work and other support services.

Attorney for personal care is someone given power of attorney by another person to make personal care decisions for that person if that person can no longer make those decisions.

Attorney for property is someone given power of attorney by another person to make decisions about that person's property if that person can no longer make those decisions.

Case managers are people who work one-on-one with clients to provide more complete, client-centred support services, particularly for people with many complex needs.

Community treatment order (CTO) is a legal order issued by a doctor and consented to by the person or the person's substitute decision-maker that sets the conditions under which the person with a serious mental health problem may live in the community.

Compliance is a client's full participation in the treatment prescribed by the doctor; for example, a person taking medication as directed and attending therapy sessions.

Concurrent disorders refer to conditions in which people have both a mental health and substance use problem.

Consumer/survivor is a term used by some people who have a mental health problem and/or who have used mental health services or programs. Some believe that they have survived a mental health problem. Others see themselves as having survived the mental health system—depending on their experiences.

Crisis is a time of danger or great difficulty. A person in crisis may feel out of control or unable to cope (e.g., the person may have difficulty sleeping, eating, paying attention or carrying on a normal routine at work, school or home).

Diversion programs are programs set up by the courts as a way to redirect clients and connect them to mental health treatment services or supports. They prevent some people from going to jail and having a criminal record.

Episode is a period when a person has symptoms of a mental health problem like depression or mania.

Forensic clients are people with mental health problems who have come into conflict with the law.

A **governing** or **regulatory college** has the legal responsibility for licensing and overseeing a specific group of health care workers. The college tries to make sure these professionals do their work properly and fairly. The college must deal with all complaints from clients. All regulated health care and social services workers in Ontario are members of colleges or governing bodies that set guidelines, rules and standards to regulate their work.

Incapable, according to the *Health Care Consent Act* and the *Substitute Decisions Act*, means that a person is unable to understand information that is needed to make certain decisions, and he or she is unable to appreciate the reasonably foreseeable consequences that making or not making a decision is likely to have.

Informed consent means making a decision knowing what your condition is, what the proposed treatment is; its possible risks, benefits and side-effects; what happens if you don't have treatment; and what other treatments are available, and then giving your consent to it.

Involuntary commitment means that a person is admitted to a hospital against his or her will for a period of time.

Mood disorder is a pattern of symptoms defined by a disturbance of mood. Bipolar disorder and depression are both mood disorders.

Naturopathic doctors are health care professionals trained to use natural methods (such as homeopathy, clinical nutrition, traditional Chinese medicine and botanical or herbal medicine) to promote healing.

Occupational therapists are regulated health professionals who help you to identify areas of your life where you are having difficulties. Their main goal is to work with you to identify what you want to do and what you need to know in terms of self-care, productivity and leisure. Learning new ways to adapt and gain new skills to live more independently and with greater happiness is the ultimate goal of occupational therapy.

Power of attorney is a legal document that a person can use to authorize another person(s) to make important decisions for him or her. There are two types of powers of attorney: for property (e.g., finances) and for personal care (e.g., health care, shelter, nutrition, hygiene, safety).

Psychosis refers to disturbances that cause someone's personality to break down. The person loses touch with reality; he or she may imagine hearing voices or seeing things or believe things that seem untrue.

Psychotherapy is a general term used to describe a form of treatment based on talking with a therapist. The purpose of psychotherapy is to relieve your distress by discussing and expressing feelings; helping you change your attitudes, behaviours and habits; and building better ways of coping.

Public Guardian and Trustee (PGT) is a government official (with a large staff) that is required by law to help people who are vulnerable by making treatment decisions for them and managing their property if they are not able to do so themselves. The PGT only steps in as a last resort, if no family member is available.

Relapse is the return of the symptoms of a mental health problem after the client appears to have improved with treatment but before the symptoms are completely gone.

Side-effects are the effects of a drug treatment that occur in addition to the desired effects. Usually side-effects are unwanted.

Sliding scale (of a cost or fee) means that the cost or fee is adjusted based on a person's income or ability to pay.

Social housing is housing that is partly paid for by the government or has rent geared to income.

Stigma refers to negative attitudes people have toward people with mental health problems, leading to prejudice and unfair and discriminatory behaviour.

Substitute decision-maker (SDM) is the person who has legal authority to make treatment or other personal care decisions for a person who is incapable.

A **support group** is a group of people who have a common interest or situation, such as the same mental health problem, who meet regularly to share ideas, feelings and community resource information.

Vocational rehabilitation specialists help people to assess their skills and abilities and develop strategies to prepare for education, training and/or employment. They also offer support to people to maintain their employment or learning situations.

Workplace accommodations are changes made to the workplace or changes in how you do the work depending on your needs. They are made in order to accommodate your special needs due to disability or handicap. Changes might involve a quieter office, more frequent breaks, time off to attend doctor's appointments, working from home, more individual supervision or direction, and so on. Accommodations are made provided that you can still do the important, central tasks of the job.

Some of the legal information contained in Appendix C and this glossary has been reproduced with permission. ©Queen's Printer for Ontario.